Pocket atlas of skeletal age

POCKET ATLAS
OF SKELETAL AGE

Dr. T. de Roo, radiologist
Central Hospital, Alkmaar,
The Netherlands

and

H. J. Schröder, radiologist
Emma Childrens Hospital, Amsterdam,
The Netherlands

MARTINUS NIJHOFF - MEDICAL DIVISION - THE HAGUE 1976

ISBN-13: 978-94-010-1425-0   e-ISBN-13: 978-94-010-1423-6
DOI: 10.1007/ 978-94-010-1423-6

A separate limited edition of this book was made financially possible by a grant
of C.G.R. Benelux.
Drawings by J. G. Hofstede - Schuurman, Nieuw Vennep.

Contents

Introduction

The reason for publishing this Pocket Atlas of Skeletal Age was, despite the existance of several standard texts on the subject, the lack of a practical guide for a rapid orientation.

The well known reference books are generally difficult to use, Having no practical divisions, these books are rather useless if a quick interpretation is needed.
The photographs in these works are often not clear, whilst frequently the skeletal age of the same child is followed, whereby small individual differences are not taken into consideration.

This Pocket Atlas is based on a large series of children. It is of handy pocket-size with a firm binding. The application of a special new technique has resulted in attractive, clear photographs, and this together with a brief, schematic text guarantees a rapid orientation for practical purposes.

Anatomy

1. Radius
2. Processus styloideus radii
3. Ulna
4. Processus styloideus ulnae
5. Os scaphoideum
6. Os lunatum
7. Os triquetrum
8. Os pisiforme
9. Os trapezium
10. Os trapezoideum
11. Os capitatum
12. Os hamatum
13. Hamulus ossis hamati
14-18. Ossa metacarpalia I-V
19-23. Phalanges proximales
24-27. Phalanges mediae
28-32. Phalanges distales
33. Ossa sesamoidea
34. Articulatio radiocarpea
35. Articulatio carpometacarpea pollicis
36. Articulationes metacarpophalangeae
37. Articulatio interphalangea proximalis indicis
38. Articulationes interphalangeae distales pollicis et indicis

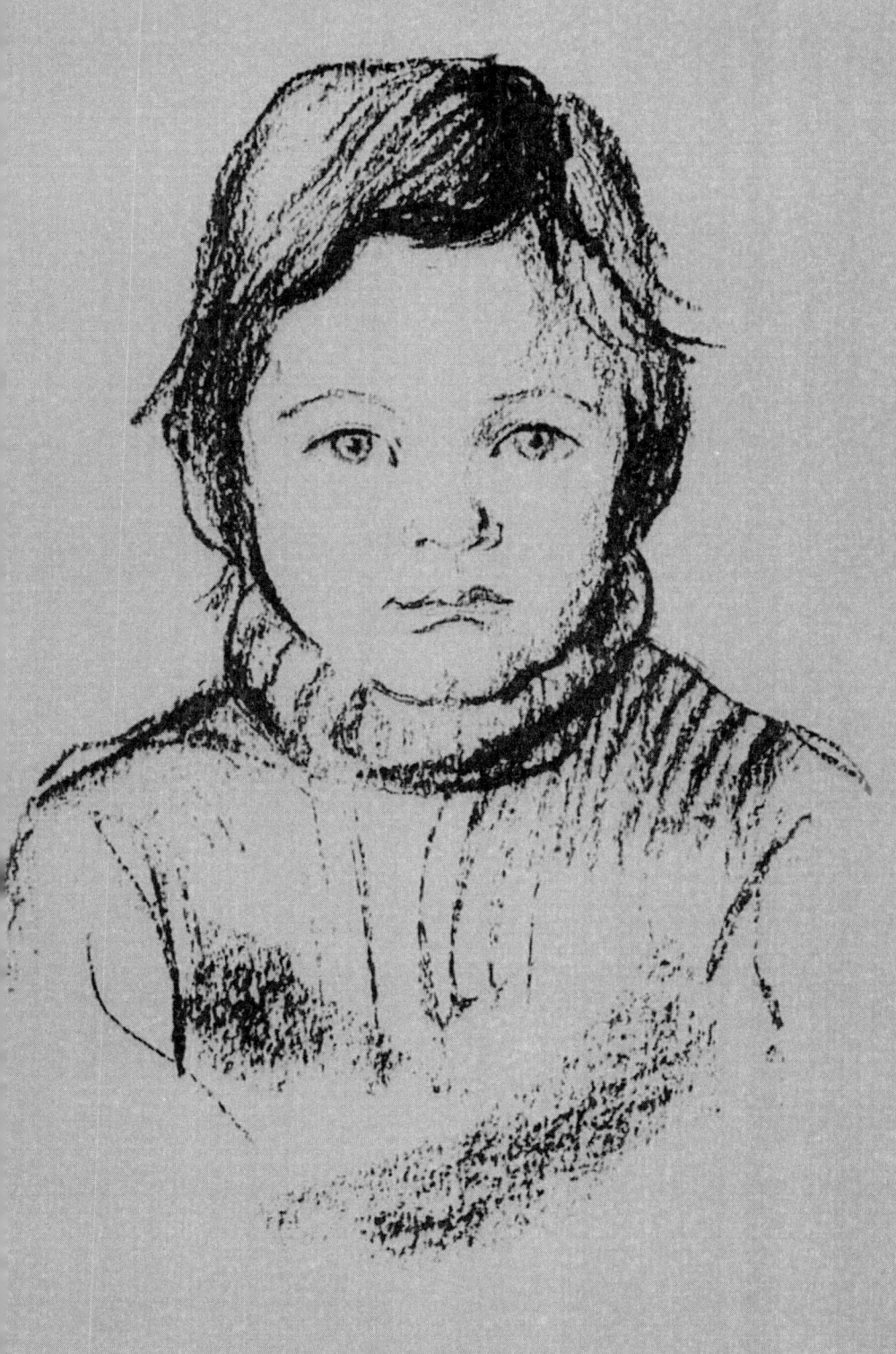

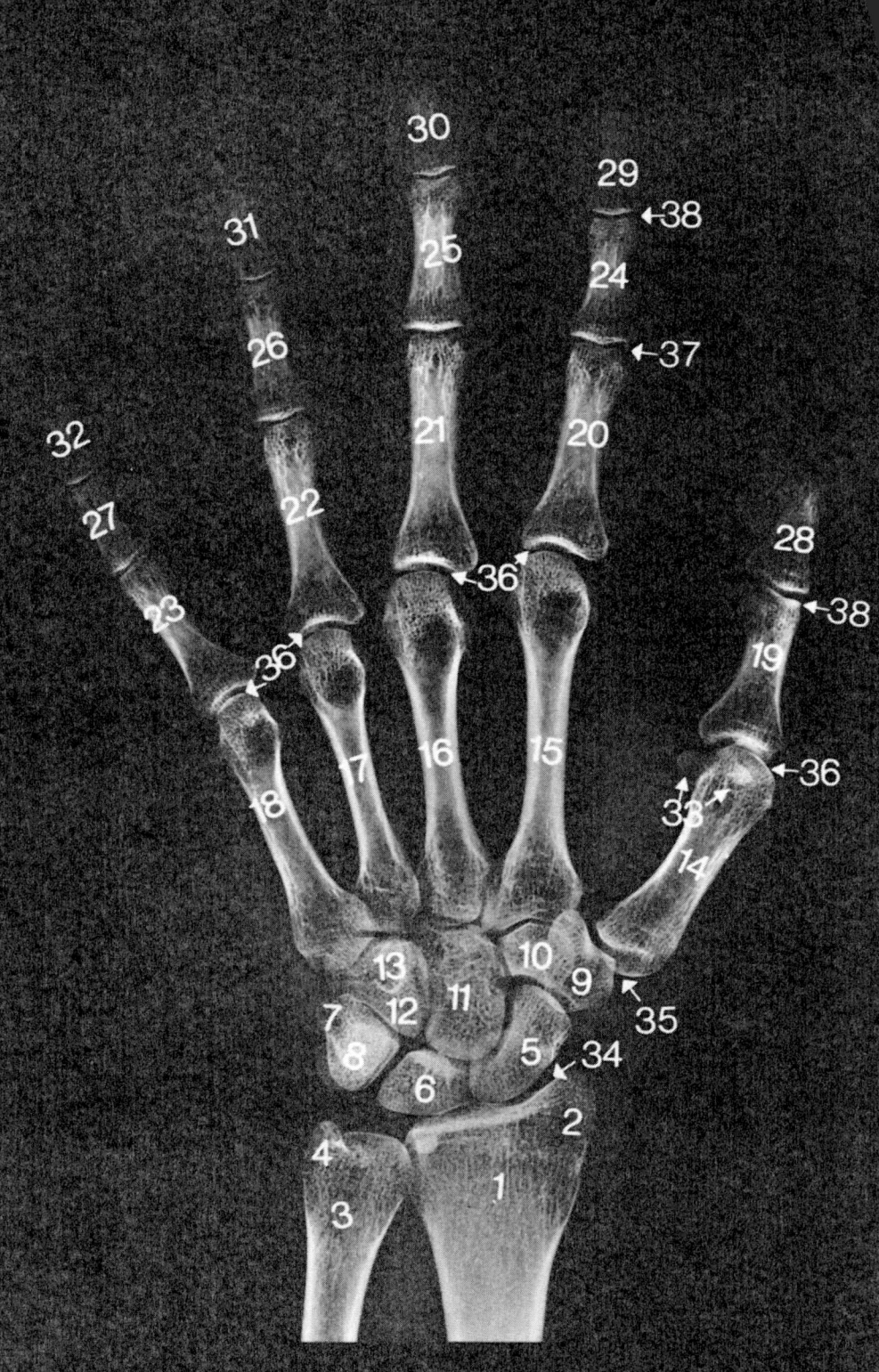

SKELETAL AGE OF BOYS

Newborn
1 month and 15 days
3 months
6 months
9 months
1 year
1 year and 3 months
1 year and 6 months
1 year and 9 months
2 years
2 years and 6 months
3 years
3 years and 6 months
4 years and 6 months
5 years
5 years and 6 months
6 years
6 years and 6 months
7 years
8 years
9 years
10 years
11 years
12 years
13 years
13 years and 6 months
14 years
15 years
16 years
17 years
18 years

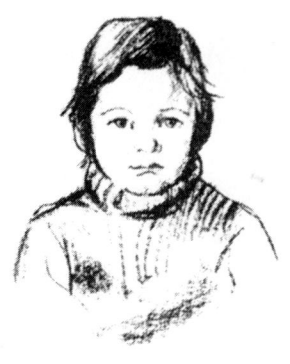

♂ Newborn

Radius and ulna: The distal ends are flared and the margins are somewhat flattened.
No ossification centers visible.
Carpal bones: No ossification centers visible.
Metacarpal bones: The shafts of the second to fifth metacarpals are slightly constricted in their middle portions. The proximal ends of the metacarpals are somewhat closer together than their distal ends and, consequently, the shafts appear to radiate out from the carpal area.
No ossification centers visible.
Phalanges: The distal ends of the proximal and middle phalanges are rounded and their proximal ends are wider and flat. No ossification centers visible.

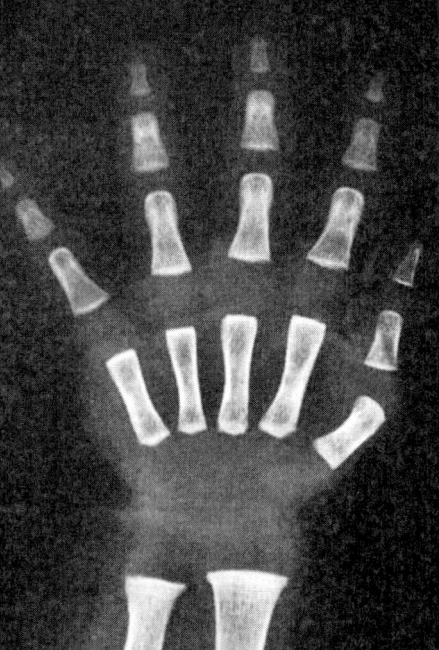

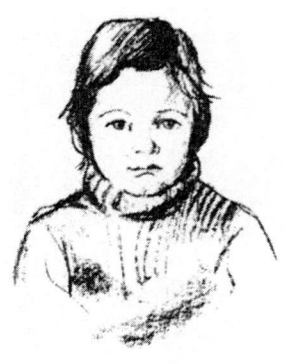

♂ 1 month and 15 days

Radius and ulna: No changes.
Carpal bones: No changes.
Metacarpal bones: The ossification centers of hamate and capitate are just visible.
Phalanges: No changes.

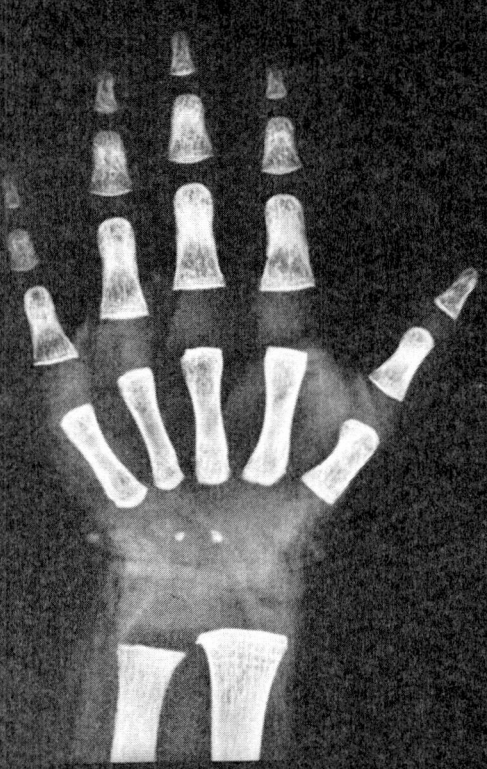

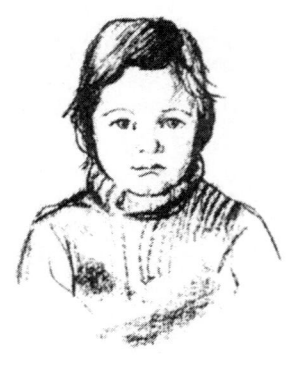

♂ 3 months

Radius and ulna: The beaklike projection on the radial side of the distal end of the ulna usually persist for several years. No ossification centers visible.

Carpal bones: A center of ossification is now visible in both the capitate and the hamate. The capitate usually reaches this stage of development slightly earlier than the hamate.

Metacarpal bones: The shafts of the metacarpals are becoming individualized in size and shape. The ends of the metacarpals have increased in width relatively more than the central portion of their shafts. The proximal ends of metacarpals II and V and the distal end of metacarpal I are more rounded than they were at birth.

The proximal or future epiphysial margin of metacarpal I is flattened. No ossification centers visible.

Phalanges: The phalanges have increased relatively more in length. Their epiphysial ends are flat and their nonepiphysial ends are rounded.

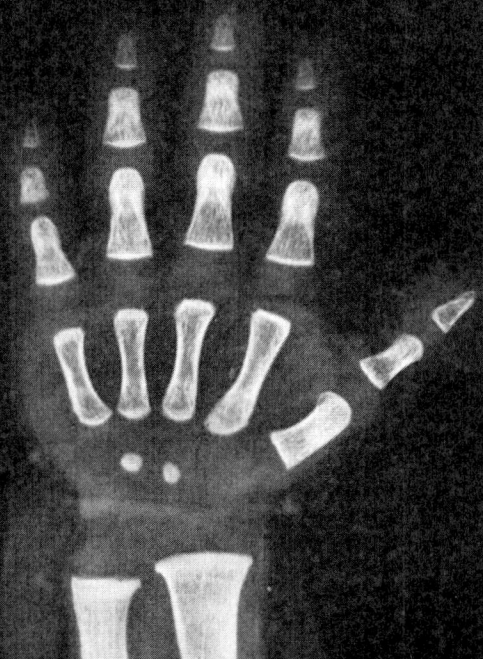

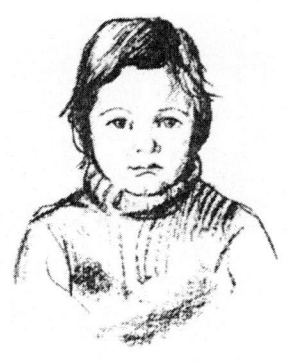

♂ 6 months

Radius and ulna: No ossification centers visible.
Carpal bones: The hamate surface of the capitate is beginning to show flattening by a reduction in the degree of its convexity. The growth of the capitate and hamate centers has brought them closer together.
Metacarpal bones: There are now individual differences in the shape and dimensions of the metacarpal shafts. No ossification centers visible.
Phalanges: No ossification centers visible.

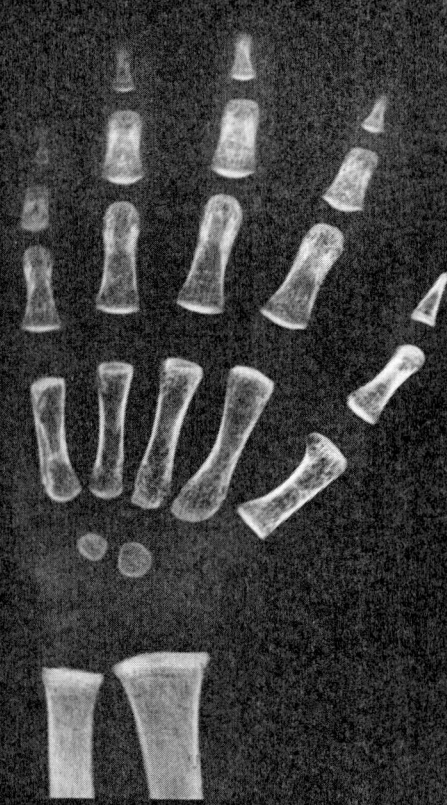

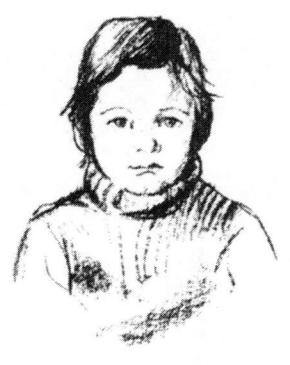

♂ 9 months

Radius and ulna: No ossification centers visible.
Carpal bones: The capitate is now larger and farther advanced in its development than the hamate.
Metacarpal bones: The base of the second, third, fourth and fifth metacarpals heve become relatively larger and more rounded. A similar change has taken place in the distal end of the first metacarpal.
Phalanges: No ossification centers visible.

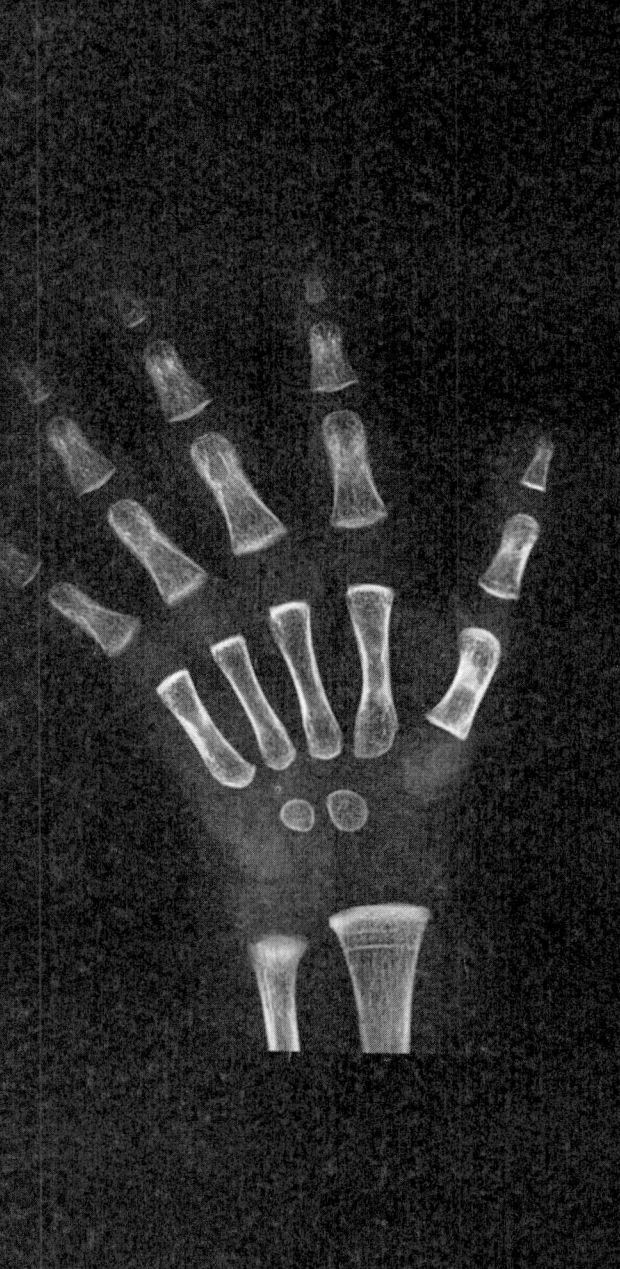

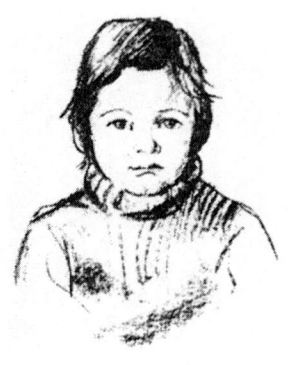

♂ 1 year

Radius and ulna: Ossification center of radius is beginning to form.
Carpal bones: The ossification centers of the capitate and hamate
have grown larger and are now close together. Some further
flattening has occured in the hamate surface of the capitate.
Matacarpal bones: No changes.
Phalanges: No changes.

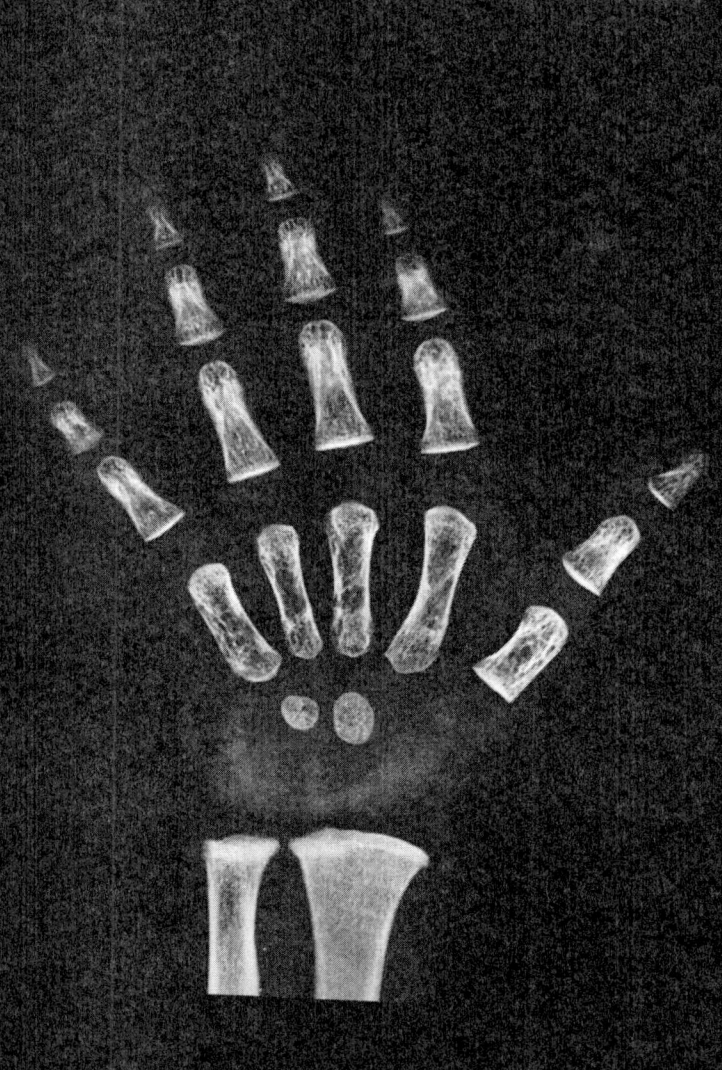

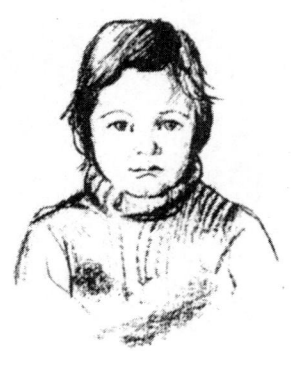

♂ 1 year and 3 months

Radius and ulna: Ossification center of the radius has enlarged.
Carpal bones: No changes.
Metacarpal bones: No changes.
Phalanges: No changes.

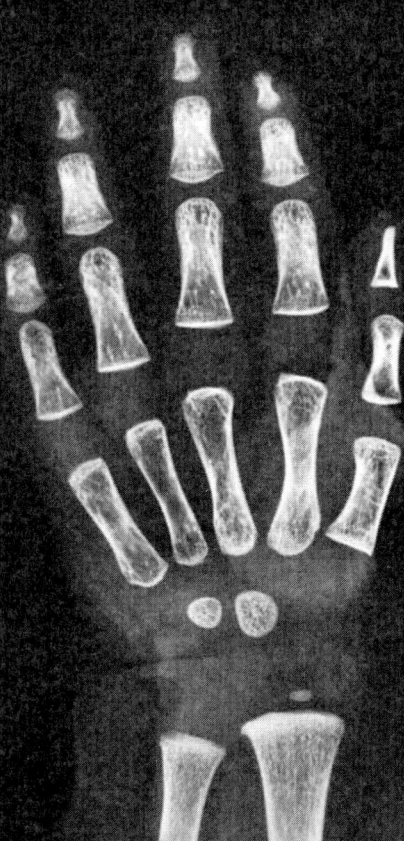

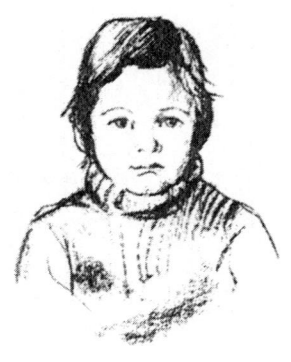

♂ 1 year and 6 months

Radius and ulna: The ulnar side of the radial epiphysis is pointed and its radial (lateral) side is thicker and convex.

Carpal bones: No changes.

Metacarpal bones: Centers of ossification are now visible in the heads of the second, third, and fourth metacarpals, in the proximal phalanges of the same fingers, and in the distal phalanx of the thumb. Ossification in these epiphyses usually appears first centrally and sub sequently extends transversely. These metacarpal epiphyses, especially that of the fourth metacarpal, are slightly advanced in their development. A small center of ossification of the base of the first metacarpal is just visible.

Phalanges: No changes.

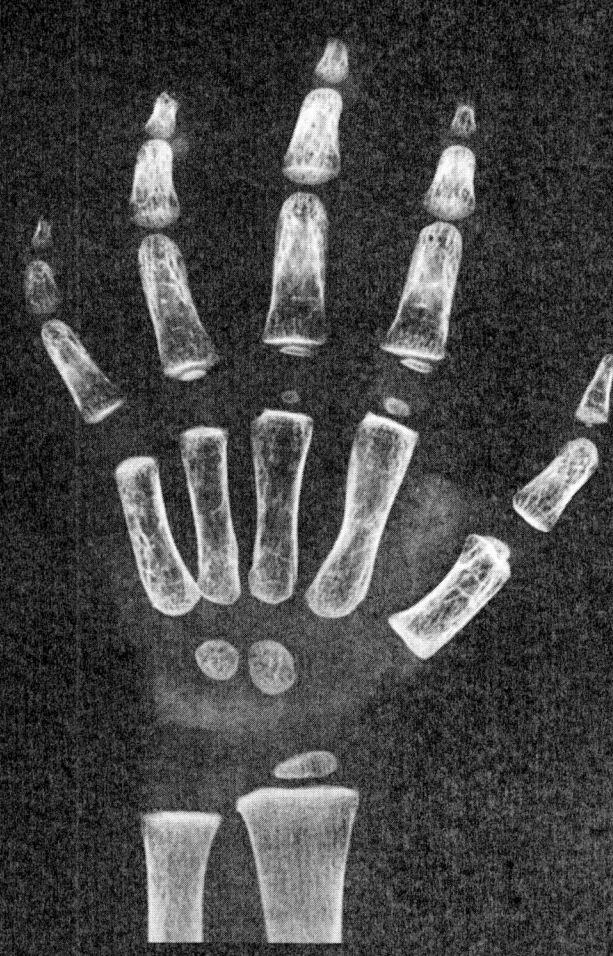

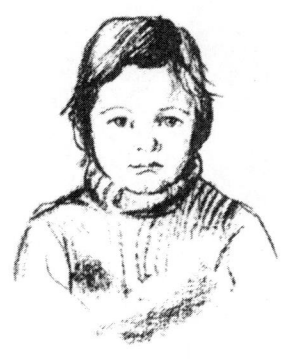

♂ 1 year and 9 months

Radius and ulna: No changes.
Carpal bones: The capitate and hamate have increased further in size.
Metacarpal bones: Ossification center of the first metacarpal has enlarged.
Phalanges: Ossification centers of the proximal phalanx of digiti V and the distal phalanges of digiti III and IV become visible.
The center of ossification of the distal phalanx of the thumb has enlarged.

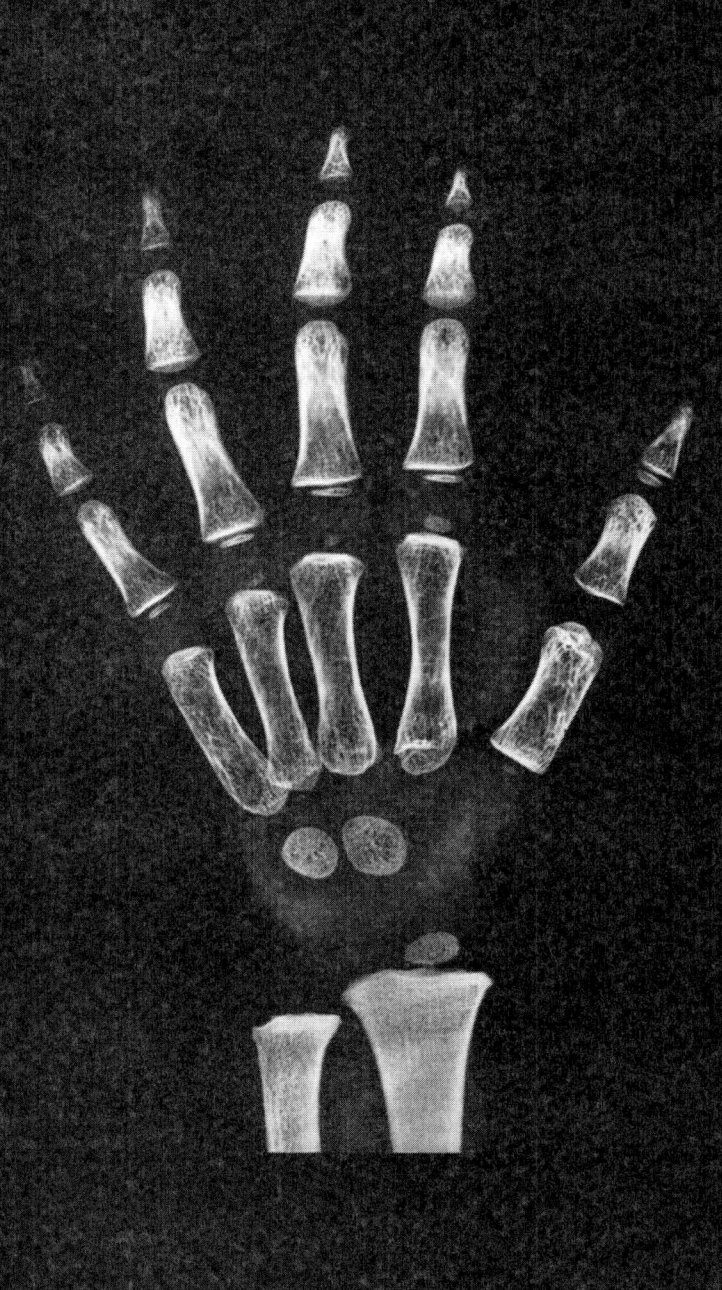

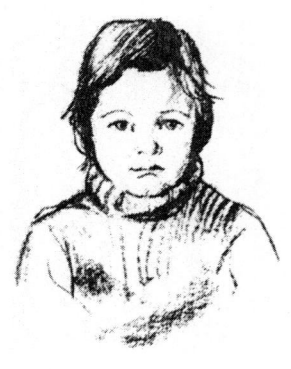

♂ 2 years

Radius and ulna: No changes.
Carpal bones: Further growth of the carpal bones.
Metacarpal bones: The ossification center of metacarpal V becomes visible.
Phalanges: The ossification centers of the epiphyses of the middle phalanges of digiti II, III and IV become visible.

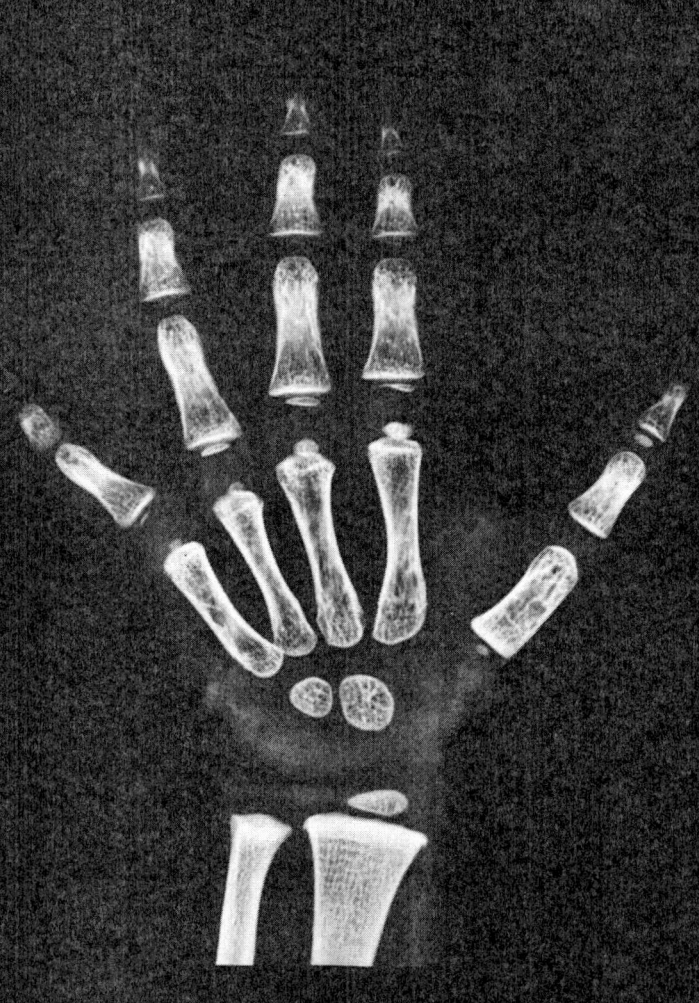

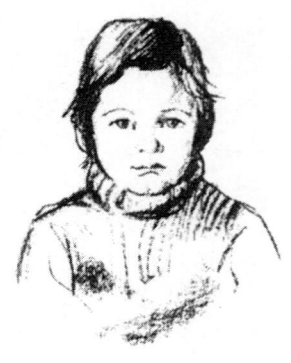

♂ 2 years and 6 months

Radius and ulna: No changes.
Carpal bones: Ossification of the triquetral bone is now visible.
Metacarpal bones: The ossification centers have enlarged and are more rounded.
Phalanges: Ossification center in the proximal phalanx of the thumb is just visible.

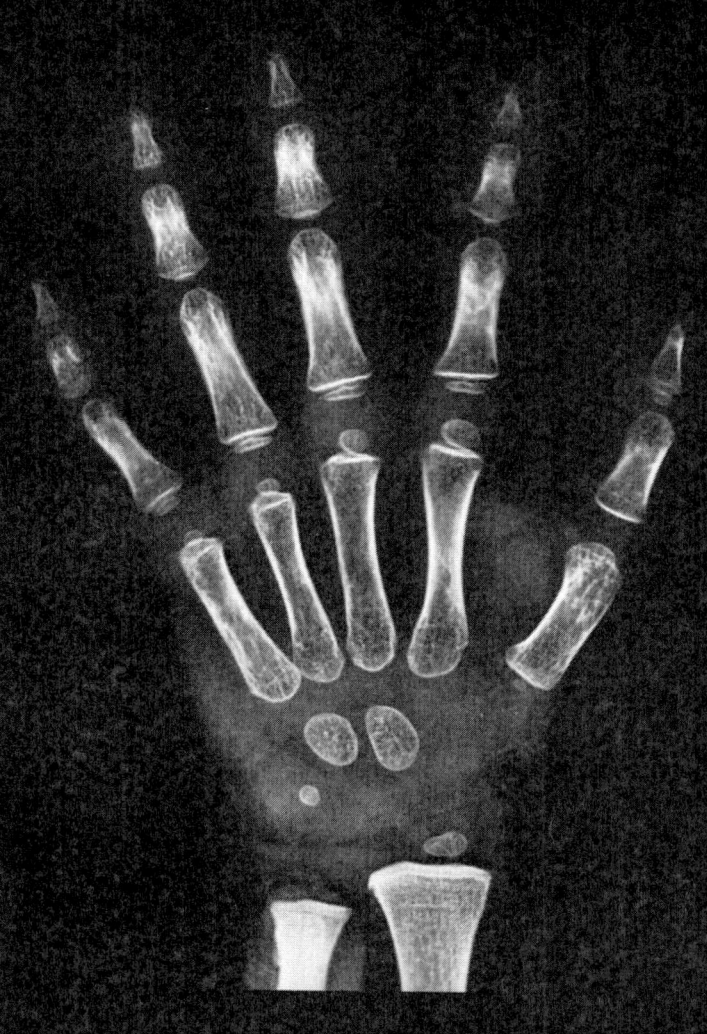

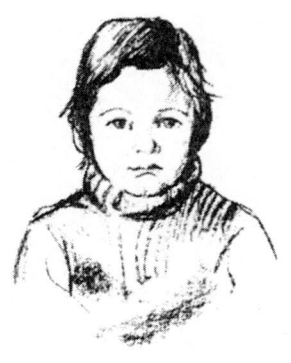

♂ 3 years

Radius and ulna: The volar and dorsal surfaces of the radial epiphysis can now be distinguished.

Carpal bones: Ossification has begun in the lunate.

Metacarpal bones: The epiphyses of the second, third, fourth and fifth metacarpals have enlarged and have become more rounded and their margins somewhat smoother.

Phalanges: Ossification is visible in all the epiphyses of the phalanges, very small in the distal phalanx of digiti II.

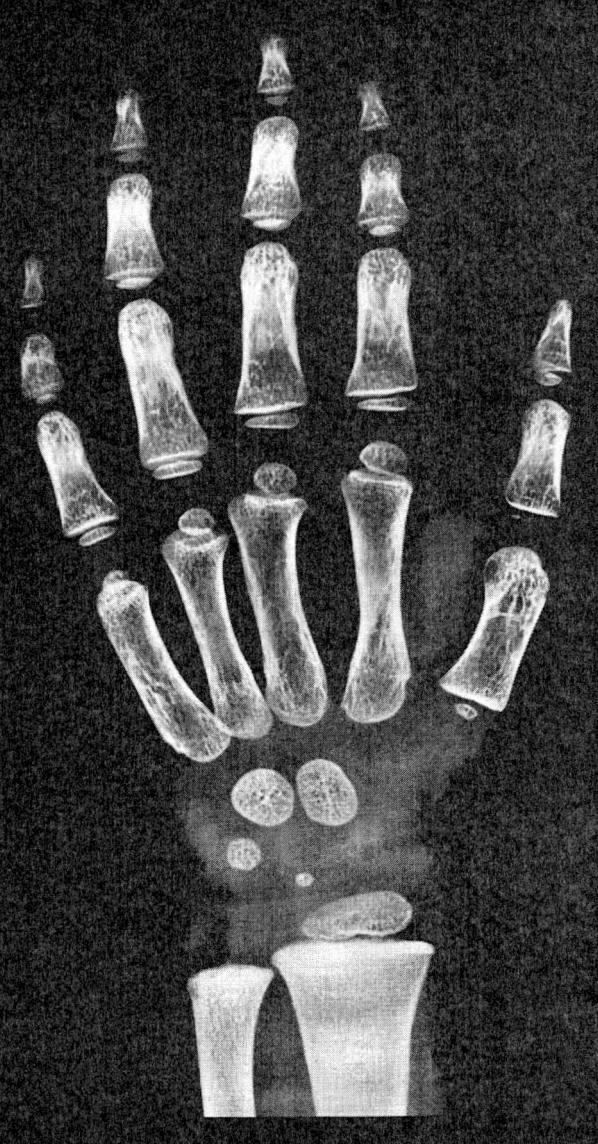

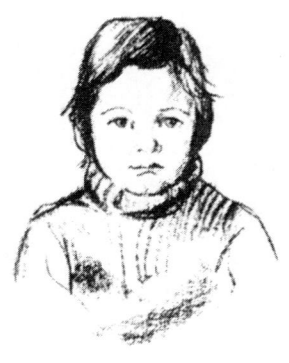

♂ 3 years and 6 months

Radius and ulna: No changes.

Carpal bones: The lunate is much advanced in its development as compared with the other bones. The approximately transverse position of its future long axis is already indicated.

Metacarpal bones: That surface of the base of the second metacarpal which will later articulate with the trapezoid has begun to flatten. The trapezoid facet makes a wide angle with the smaller capitate facet, which forms the remainder of the proximal border of the shaft.

Phalanges: The epiphyses of the distal phalanges of the second and fifth fingers are now clearly visible. The corresponding epiphyses of the third and fourth fingers are now disc shaped and their margins are smooth.

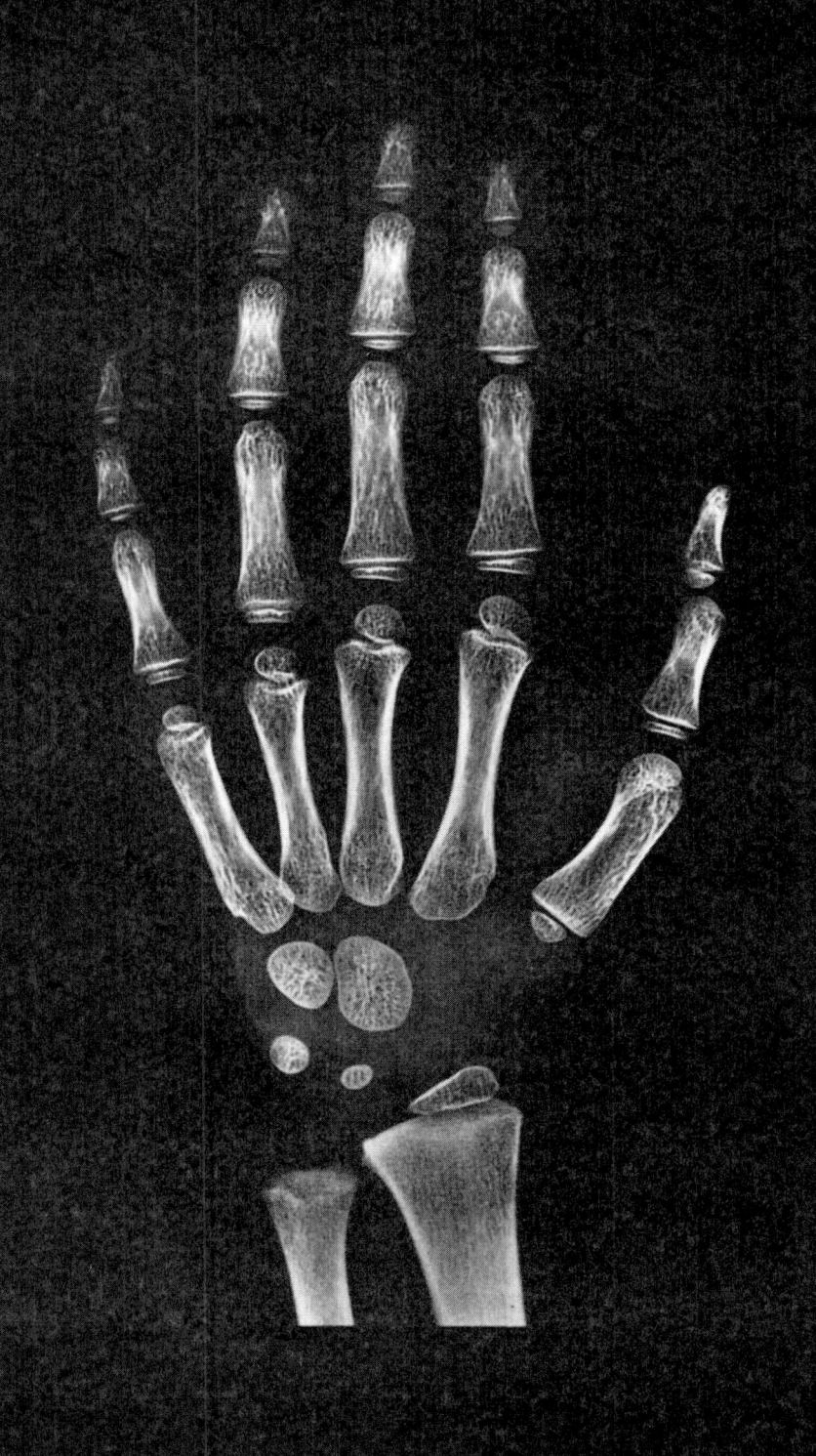

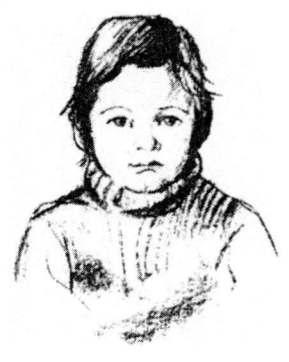

♂ 4 years and 6 months

Radius and ulna: Growth of the epiphyse of the radius. The volar and dorsal surfaces are more distinguished.

Carpal bones: Ossification center of the trapezium is visible. The long axis of the triquetral bone is clearly formed.

Metacarpal bones: No changes.

Phalanges: The epiphyses of the middle phalanges of digiti II, III and IV are now slightly more than half as wide as their shafts.

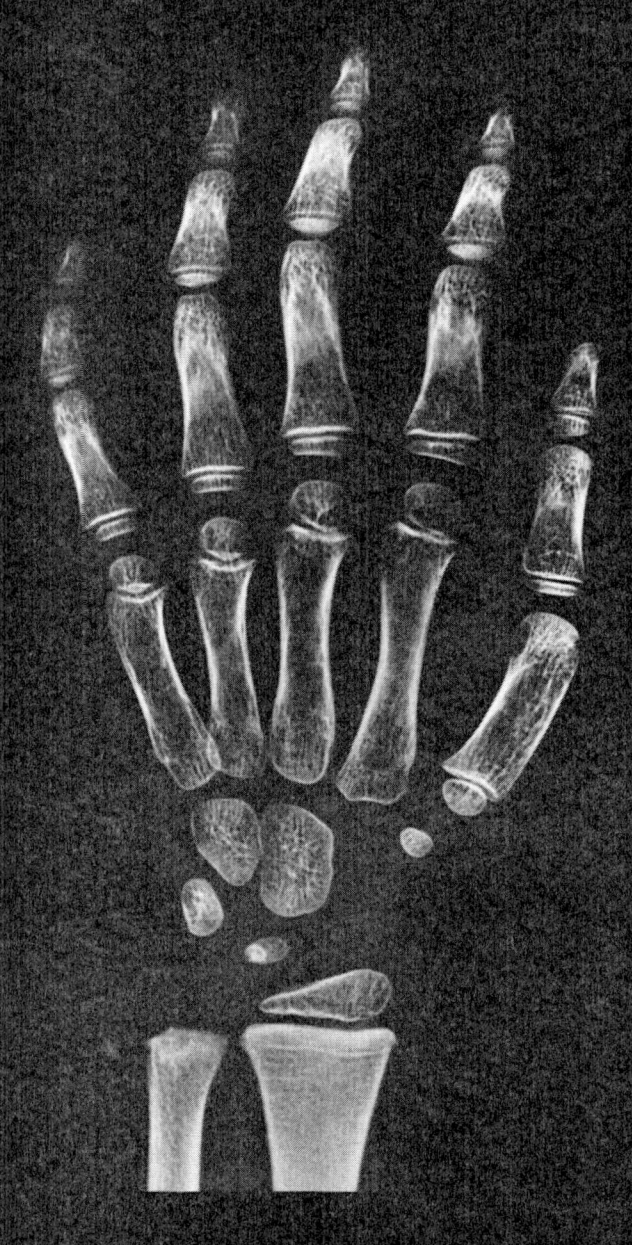

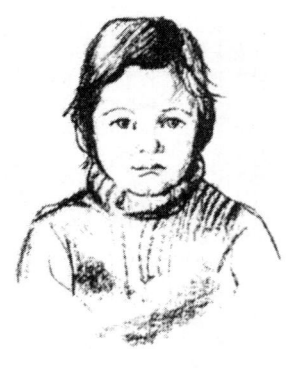

♂ 5 years

Radius and ulna: No changes.

Carpal bones: Both a lunate and a hamate facet can now be distinguished on the triquetral. Its free surface remains convex. Ossification of the trapezoïd is visible.

Metacarpal bones: The epiphysis of the first metacarpal is now more than half as wide as its metaphysis.

Phalanges: No changes.

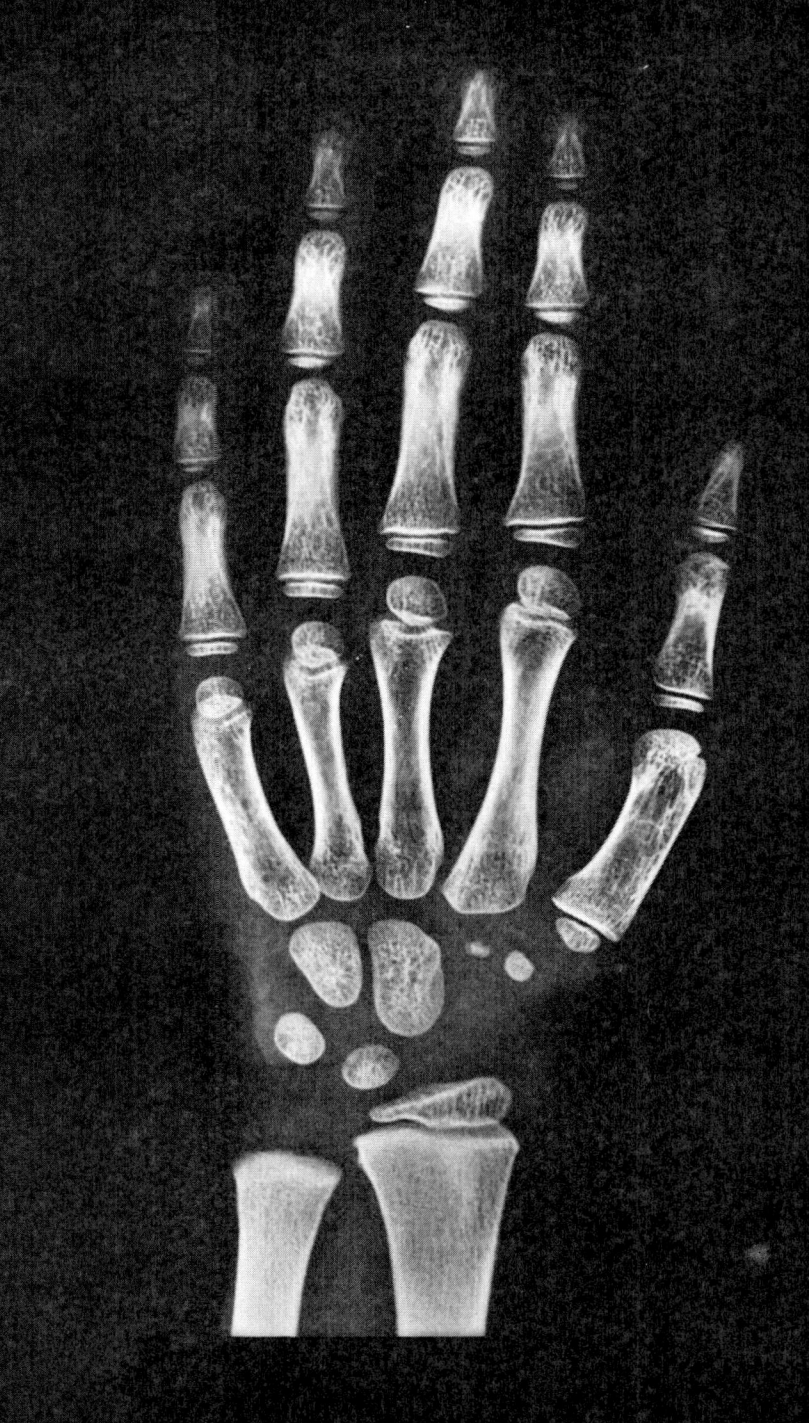

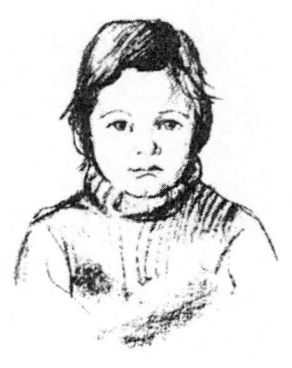

♂ 5 years and 6 months

Radius and ulna: No changes.
Carpal bones: Ossification center of the scaphoïd is visible.
Metacarpal bones: The trapezoïd facet of the proximal end of the second metacarpal is now slightly concave.
Phalanges: The epiphysis of the distal phalanges are now as wide as their shafts.

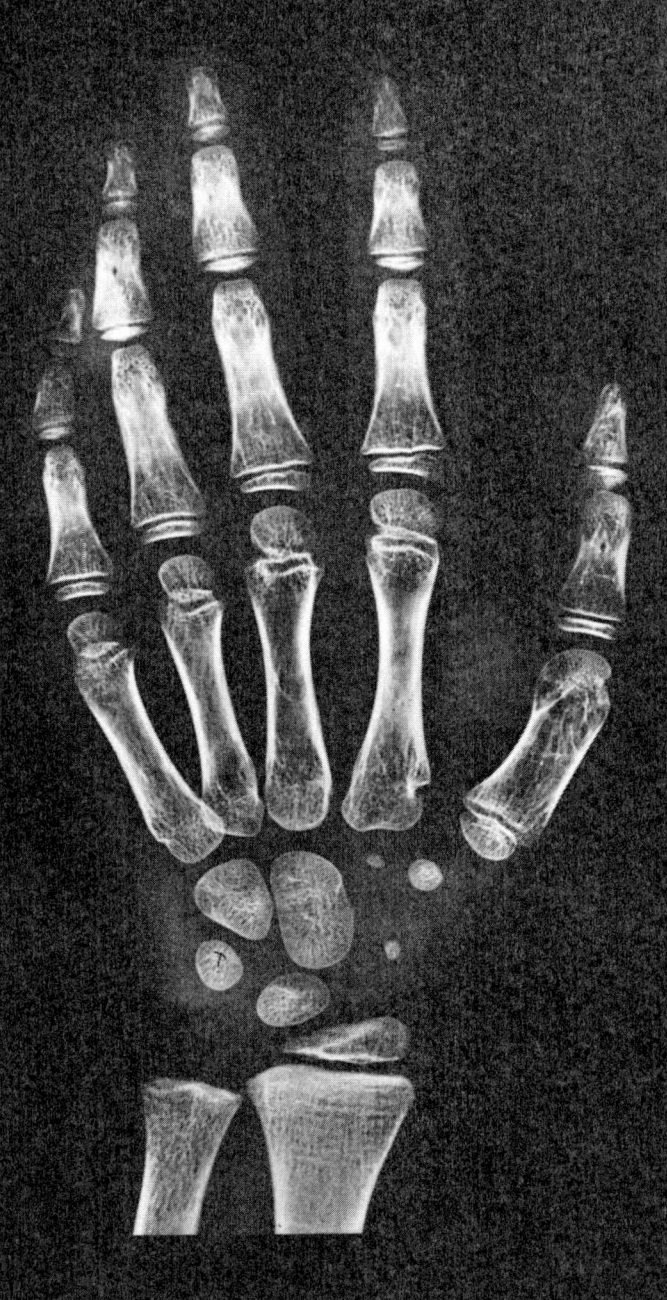

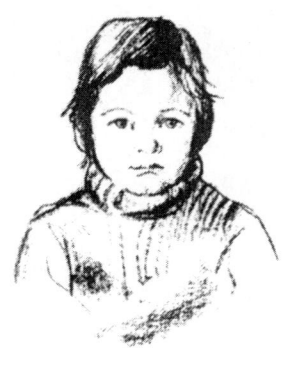

♂ 6 years

Radius and ulna: Ossification of the ulna epiphysis has begun.
Carpal bones: The capitate and hamate have increased further in size and their margins now show beginning regional differentiation. The spaces between the hamate and triquetral, capitate and lunate and lunate and radial epiphysis have been further reduced.
The surface of the trapezium adjacent to the epiphysis of the first metacarpal has begun to flatten.
Metacarpal bones: The base of the second metacarpal is now distinctly indented in the region which will later articulate with the trapezoïd.
Phalanges: No changes.

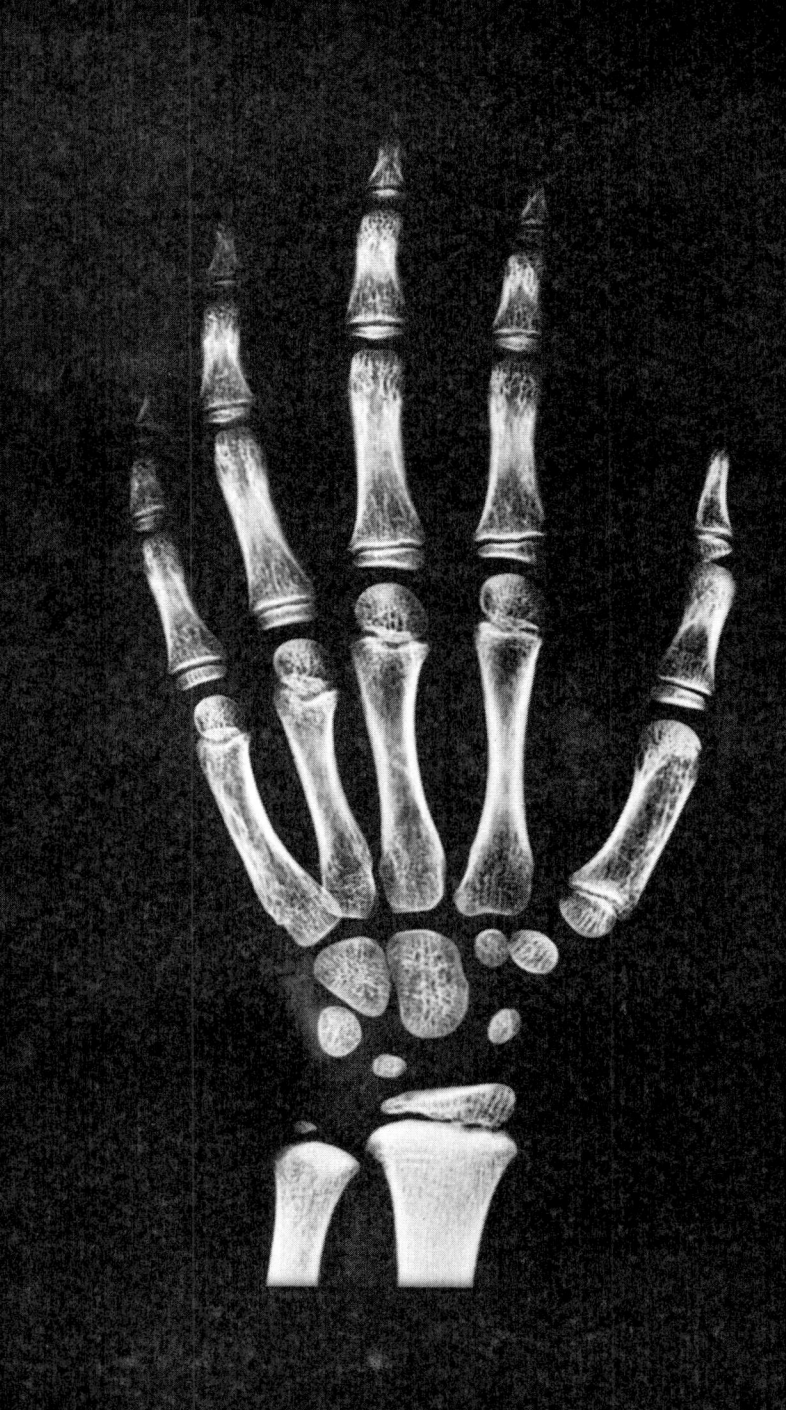

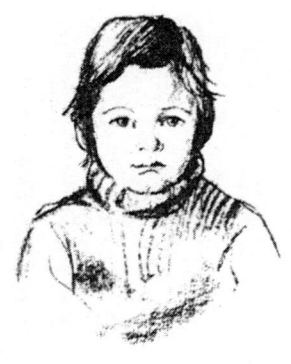

♂ 6 years and 6 months

Radius and ulna: The part of the radial epiphysis from which the styloid process develops is beginning to enlarge. Growth of the ulnar epiphyse.

Carpal bones: The distinct curved white line which occupied part of the distal margin of the lunate represents a portion of its volar surface. The triquetral has become more elongated, its ulnar margin somewhat less convex, and its hamate and lunate margins further flattened.

The trapezium, trapezoïd and scaphoïd have enlarged.

Metacarpal bones: No changes.

Phalanges: No changes.

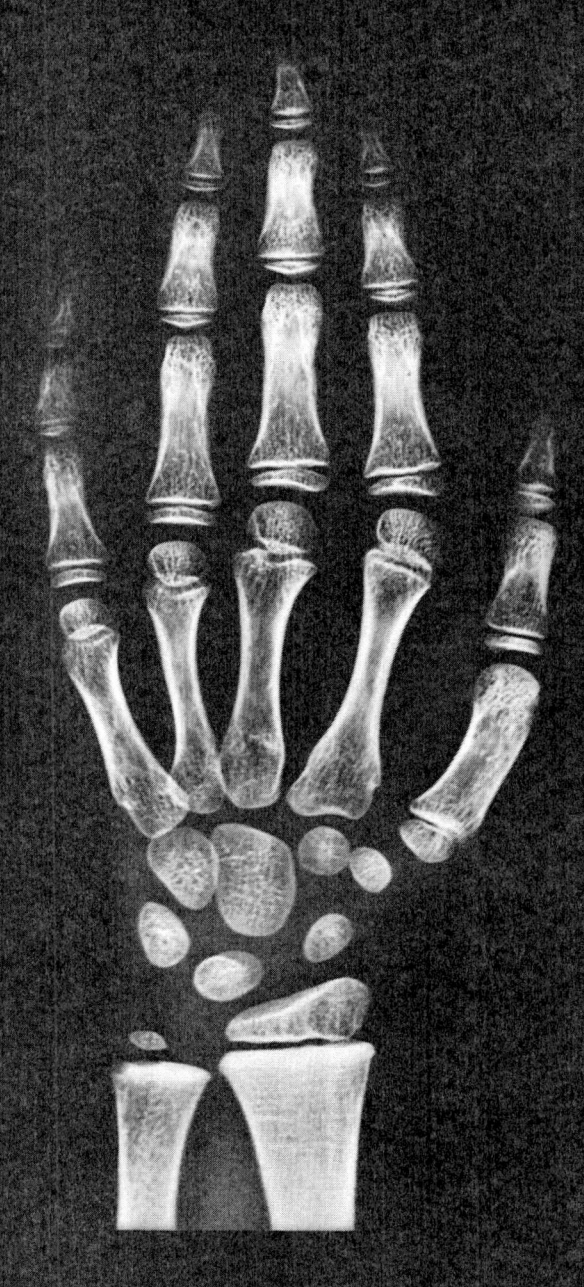

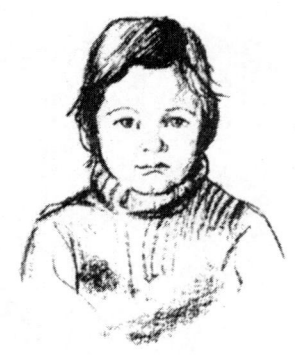

♂ 7 years

Radius and ulna: Further growth of the ulnar epiphyse.
Carpal bones: No changes.
Metacarpal bones: No changes.
Phalanges: No changes.

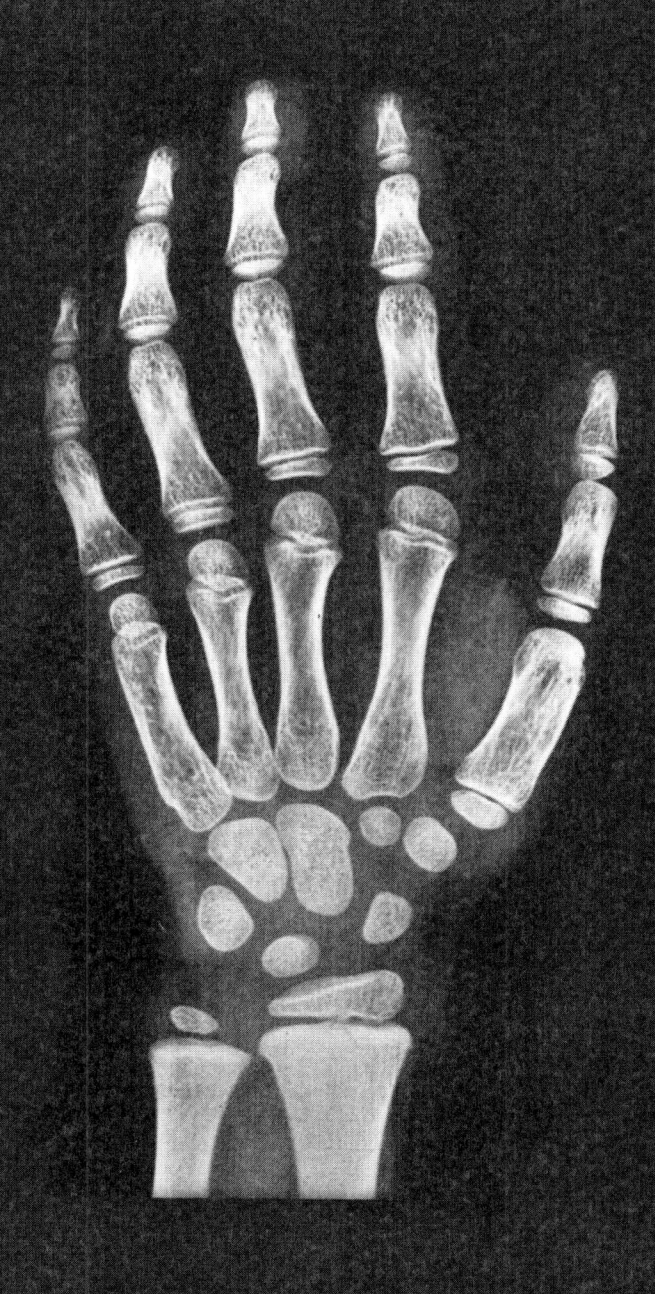

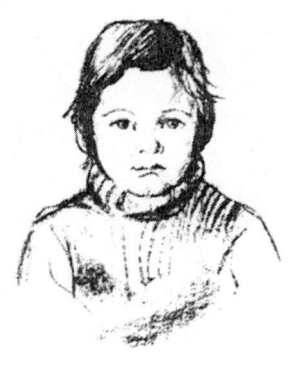

♂ 8 years

Radius and ulna: The ulnar epiphysis has extended radialward.
Carpal bones: The spaces between all the carpal bones have been further reduced.
Metacarpal bones: No changes.
Phalanges: No changes.

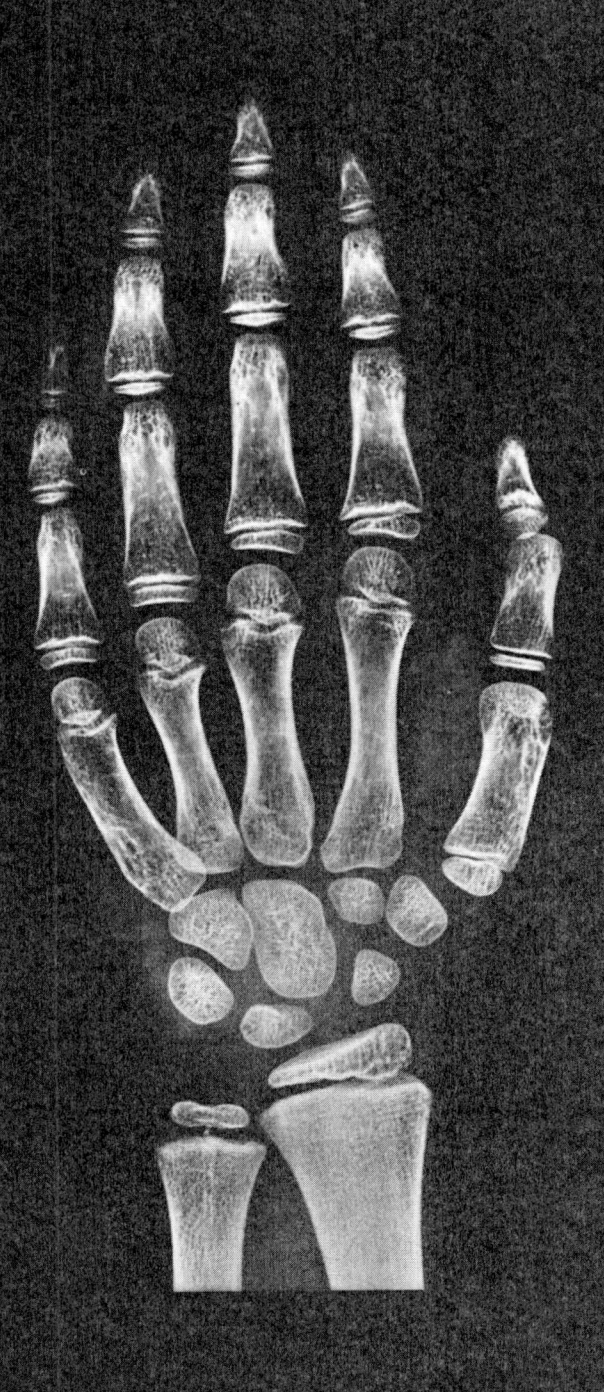

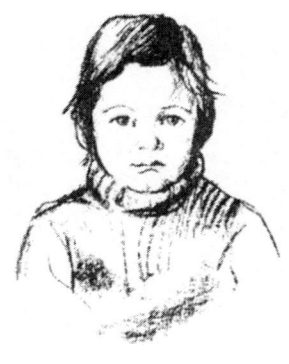

♂ 9 years

Radius and ulna: The styloïd process of the epiphysis of the ulna is beginning to appear.

Carpal bones: The white lines adjacent to the metacarpal surface of the hamate, capitate and trapezoïd mark apart of their respective volar margins.

The trapezium and trapezoïd will overlap.

As the scaphoïd has elongated its capitate surface has become somewhat less convex.

Metacarpal bones: The concavity of the base of the second metacarpal has become more pronounced.

Phalanges: No changes.

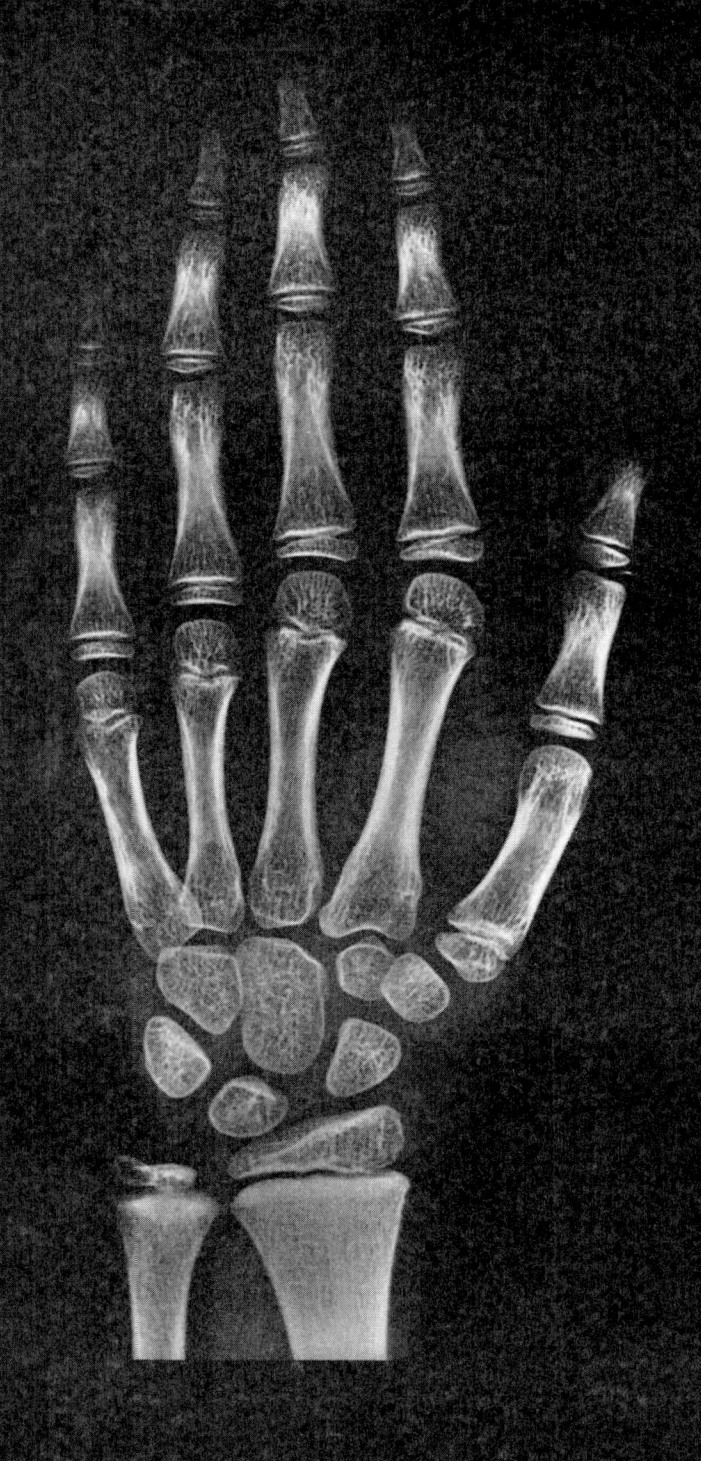

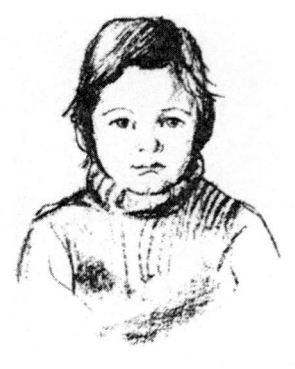

♂ 10 years

Radius and ulna: Further growth of styloïd process of the ulna.
Carpal bones: A part of the outline of the volar margin of the capitate
surface of the scaphoïd can now be seen as a rather heavy white line.
A sligth indentation has appeared in the distal surface of the
trapezium in the area of its future articulation with the first
metacarpal. Its scaphoïd surface has begun to flatten. A similar but
less marked flattening is visible in the surface of the trapezoïd which
is adjacent to the scaphoïd.
Indentation occurs in the radial site of the capitate.
A part of the volar margin of the triquetral bone can now be seen.
Ossification has begun in the pisiforme.
Metacarpal bones: The epiphysis of the first metacarpal has a sligth
indentation on its future articular surface.
Phalanges: The ends of the distal phalanges become as wide as their
base.

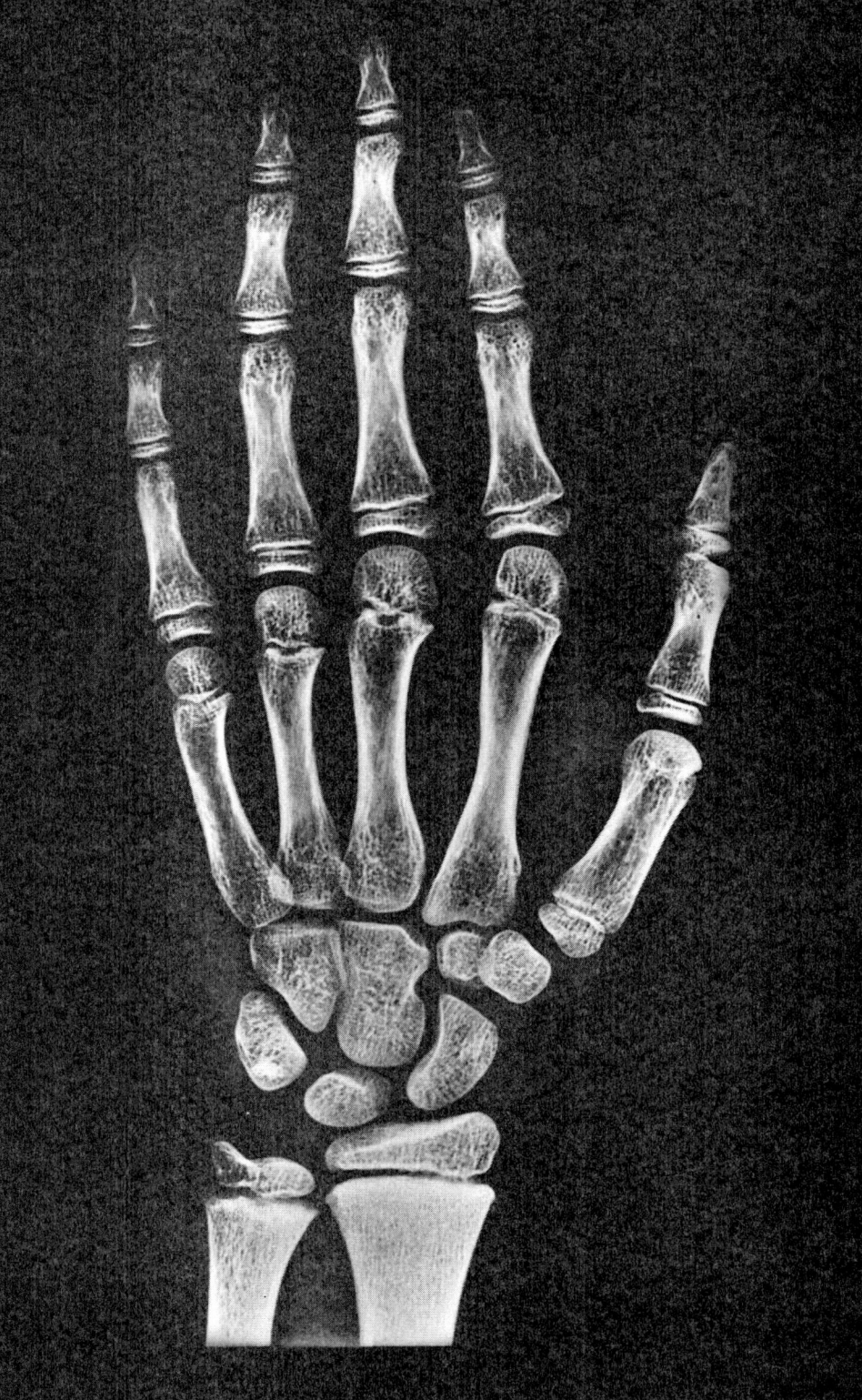

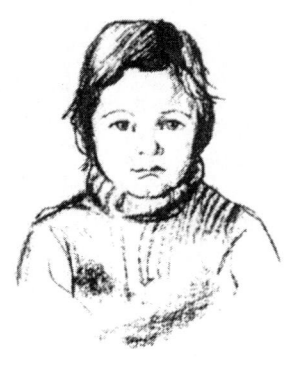

♂ 11 years

Radius and ulna: No changes.

Carpal bones: The distal tip of the hamulus of the hamate is just becoming discernible. The future scaphoid and radial articular surfaces of the lunate now are beginning to be defined.

The distal margin of the scaphoid is now somewhat flattened and its capitate articular surface dinstinctly concave. The pisiform is now more distinct.

Reducing of the spaces between the carpal bones.

Metacarpal bones: The faint white lines which are more distinct along the ulnar and proximal margins of the epiphysis of the second metacarpal outline a portion of the volar surface of that epiphysis. The process of reciprocal shaping of the proximal surface of this epiphysis to its shaft is slightly farther advanced than the same process in the other metacarpals.

Phalanges: No changes.

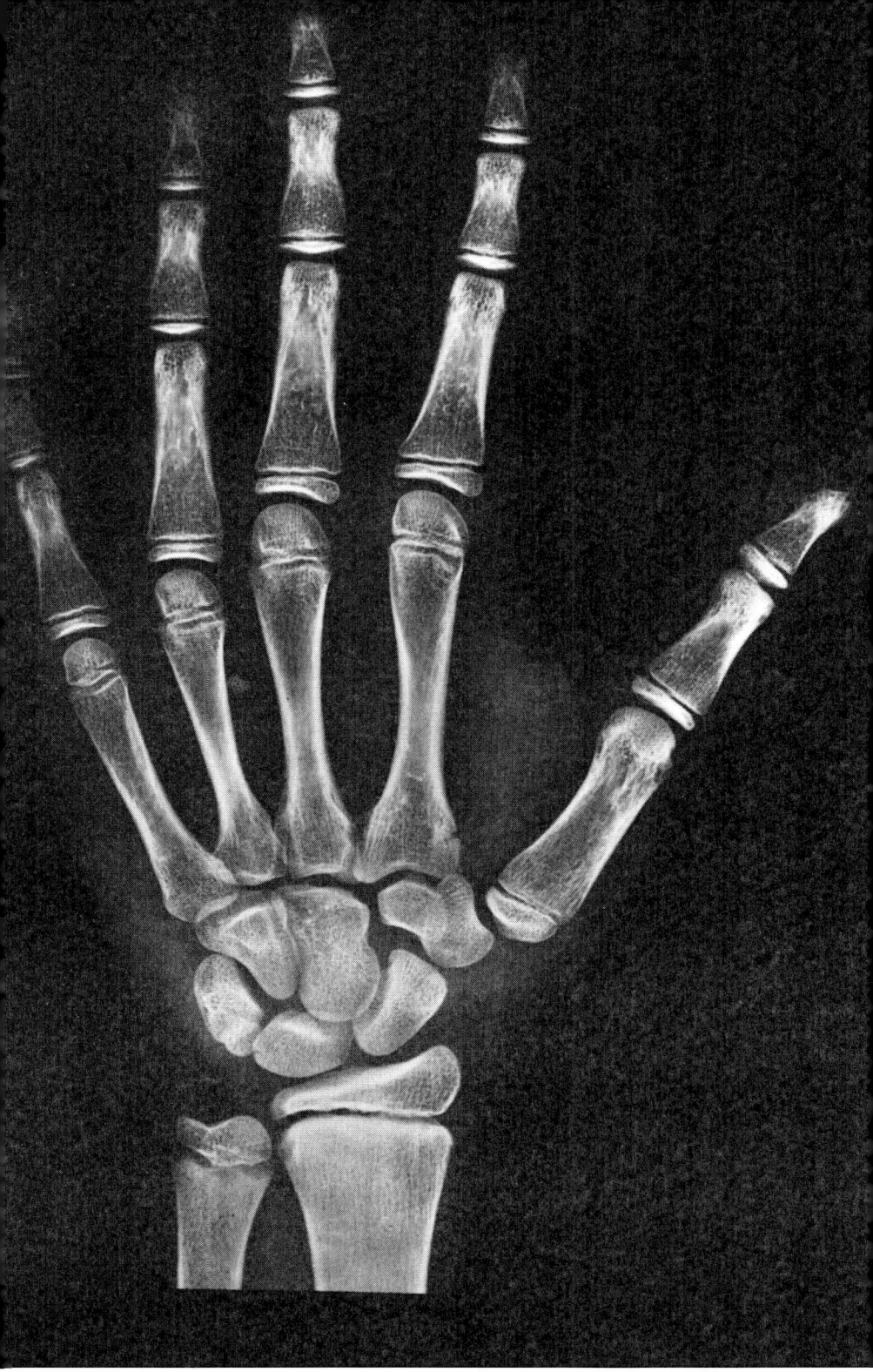

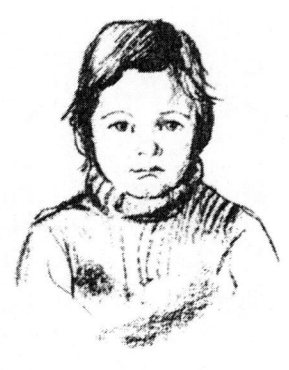

♂ 12 years

Radius and ulna: No changes.
Carpal bones: Further reducing of the spaces between the carpal bones. The capitate surface of the scaphoid now sligthly overlaps the adjacent portion of the capitate.
Metacarpal bones: No changes.
Phalanges: No changes.

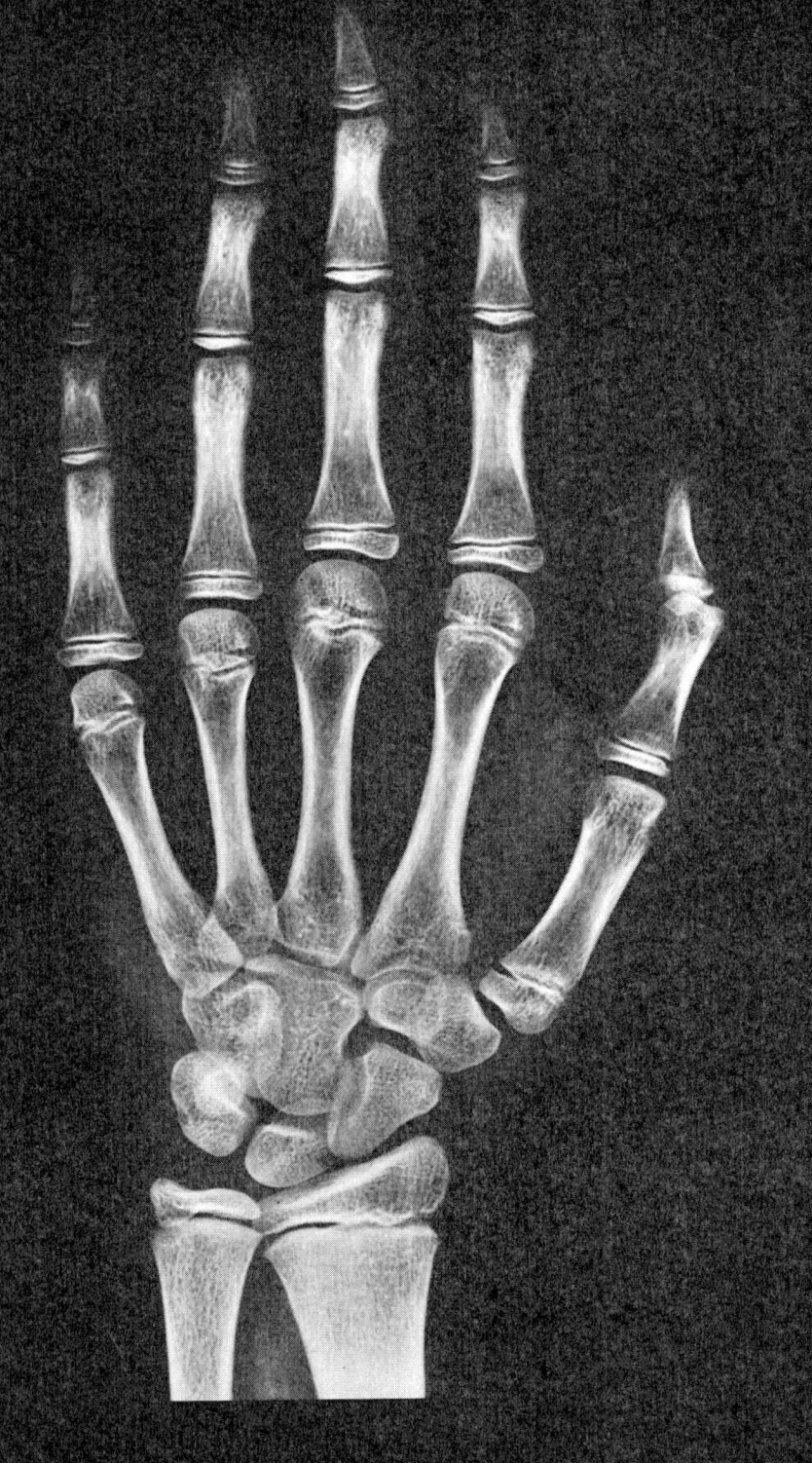

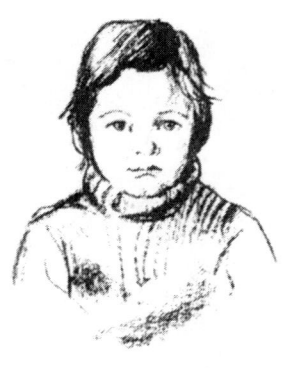

♂ 13 years

Radius and ulna: The styloïd process of the ulna has become more distinct.

Carpal bones: No changes.

Metacarpal bones: The epiphyses of the second to fifth metacarpals are now as wide as the adjacent margins of their shafts.

The ossification center of the sesamoïd in the tendon of the adductor pollicis is now visible, just medial to the head of the first metacarpel.

Phalanges: The epiphyses of the proximal phalanges of the second, third, fourth, and fifth fingers have increased somewhat in thickness and their radial margins end in distally directed tips.

The epiphysis of the middle phalanx of the fifth finger is now as wide as its shaft. The tips of the epiphyses of the distal phalanges of the second to fifth fingers are bent sligthly distally and the distal ends of the corresponding middle phalanges are now slightly concave.

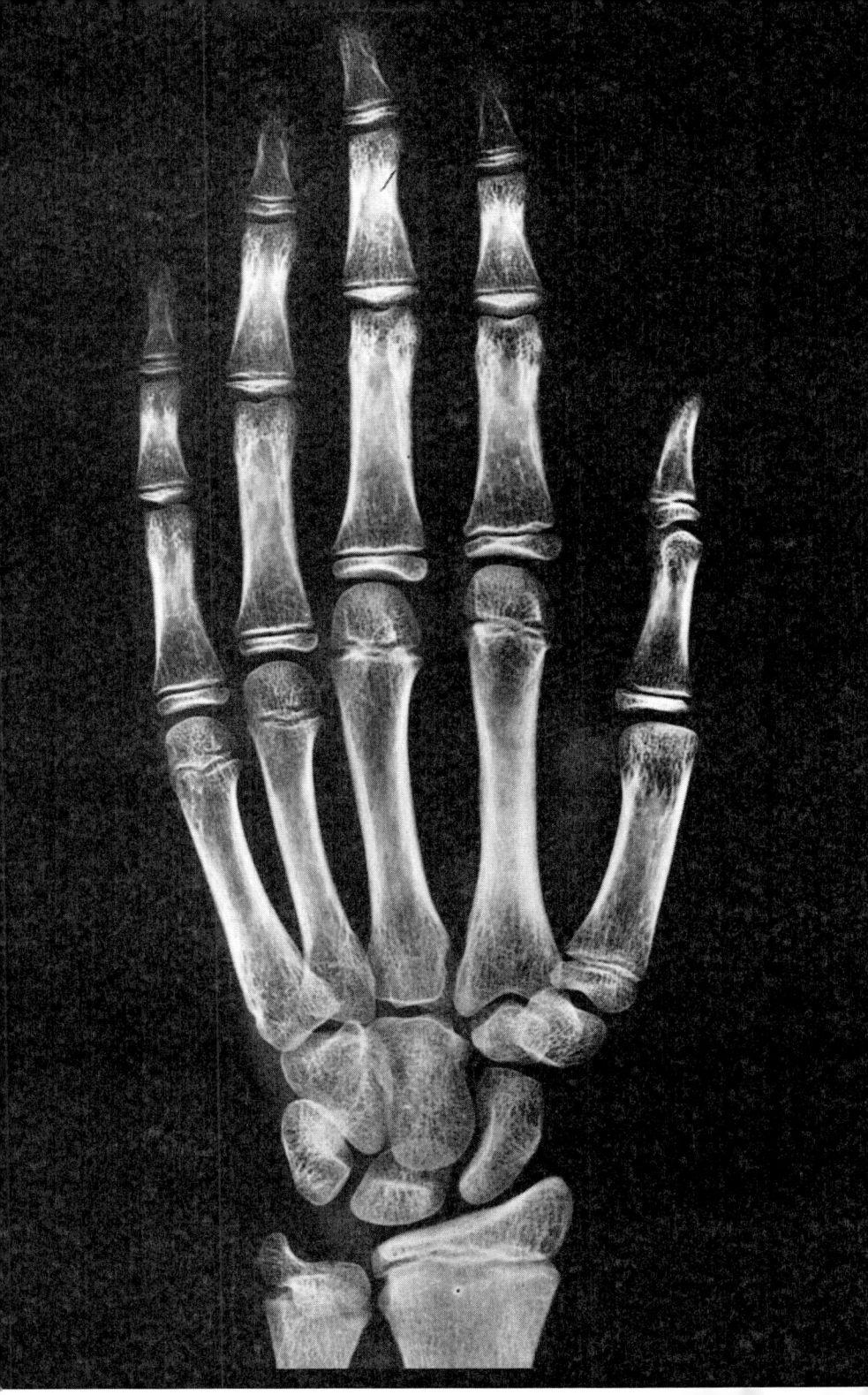

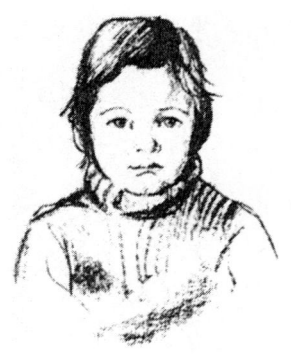

♂ 13 years and 6 months

Radius and ulna: The proximal margins of the radial and ulnar epiphyses have adjusted further to the shape of the adjacent surface of their shafts. The ulnar articular surface of the radius is now flattened.
Carpal Bones: The complete outline of the hamulus of the hamate can now be seen distinctly. The scaphoid is more elongated. The surface of the trapezium which articulates with the first metacarpal has become more concave and the proximal borders of its dorsal and volar surfaces are now distinguishable. The articular surfaces of the trapezoid are now well differentiated.
Metacarpal bones: The epiphyses of all the metacarpals are now clearly as wide as their shafts, and these adjacent margins conform closely in shape. Growth of the sesamoid of the M. adductor pollicis.
Phalanges: All of the proximal epiphyses have begun to cap their shafts.

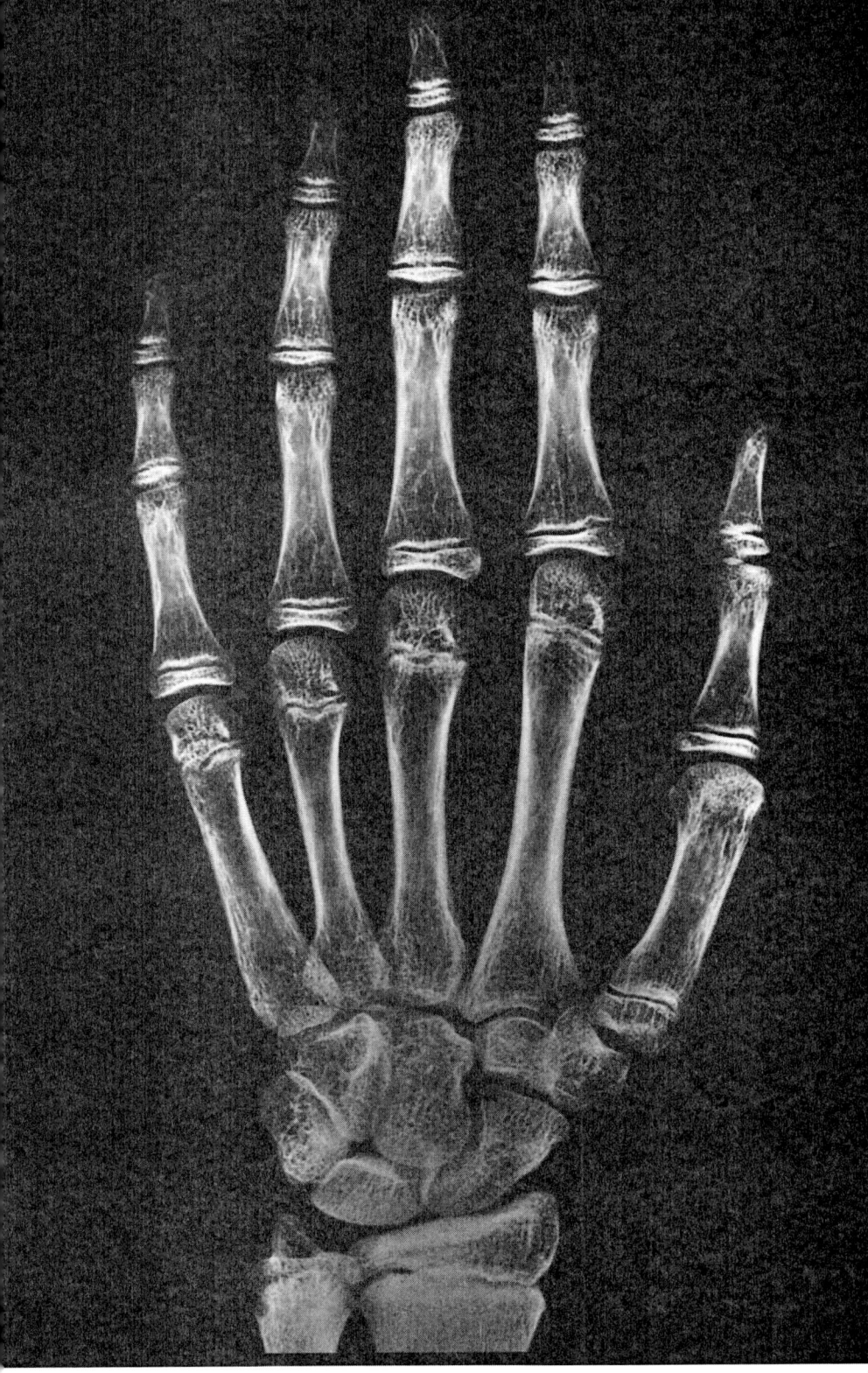

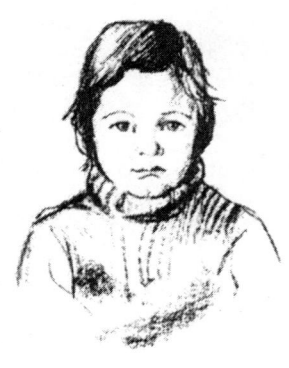

♂ 14 years

Radius and ulna: The epiphysis of the radius has become to cap its shaft.

Carpal bones: No changes.

Metacarpal bones: No changes.

Phalanges: The epiphyses of the phalanges of the second, third, fourth and fifth fingers have become to cap their shafts.

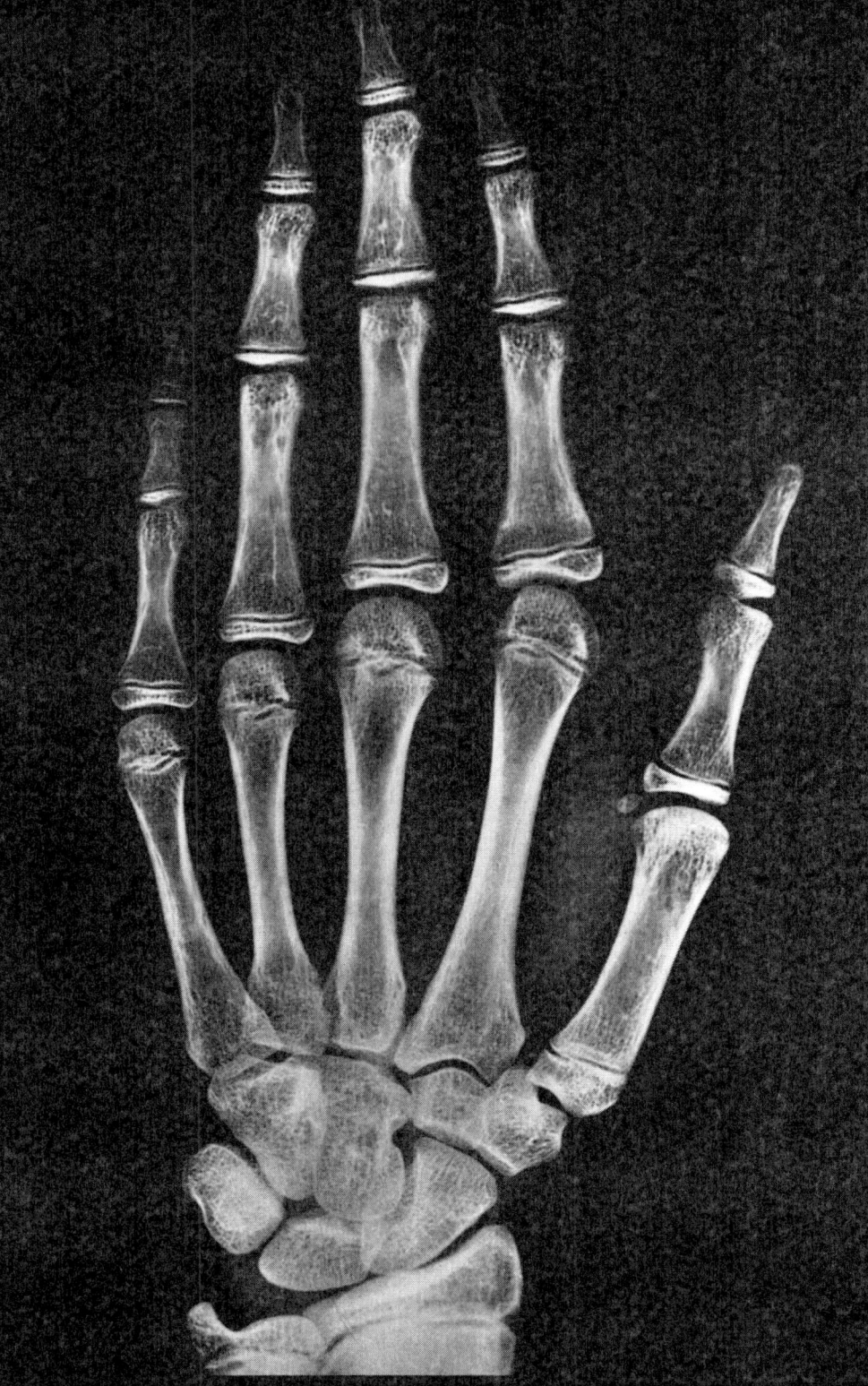

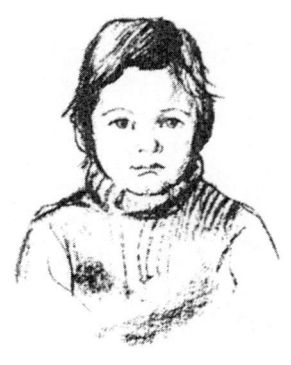

♂ 15 years

Radius and ulna: The epiphysis of the radius has capped its shaft. The epiphysis of the ulna is now as wide as its shaft and follows its contour closely. The spaces which separated the radial and ulnar epiphyses from their shafts have been somewhat reduced.
Carpal bones: No changes.
Metacarpal bones: Fusion starts in the epiphysis of metacarpale I. There are two more sesamoid bones visible in the thumb.
Phalanges: Fusion starts in the epiphysis of the distal phalanx of the thumb.

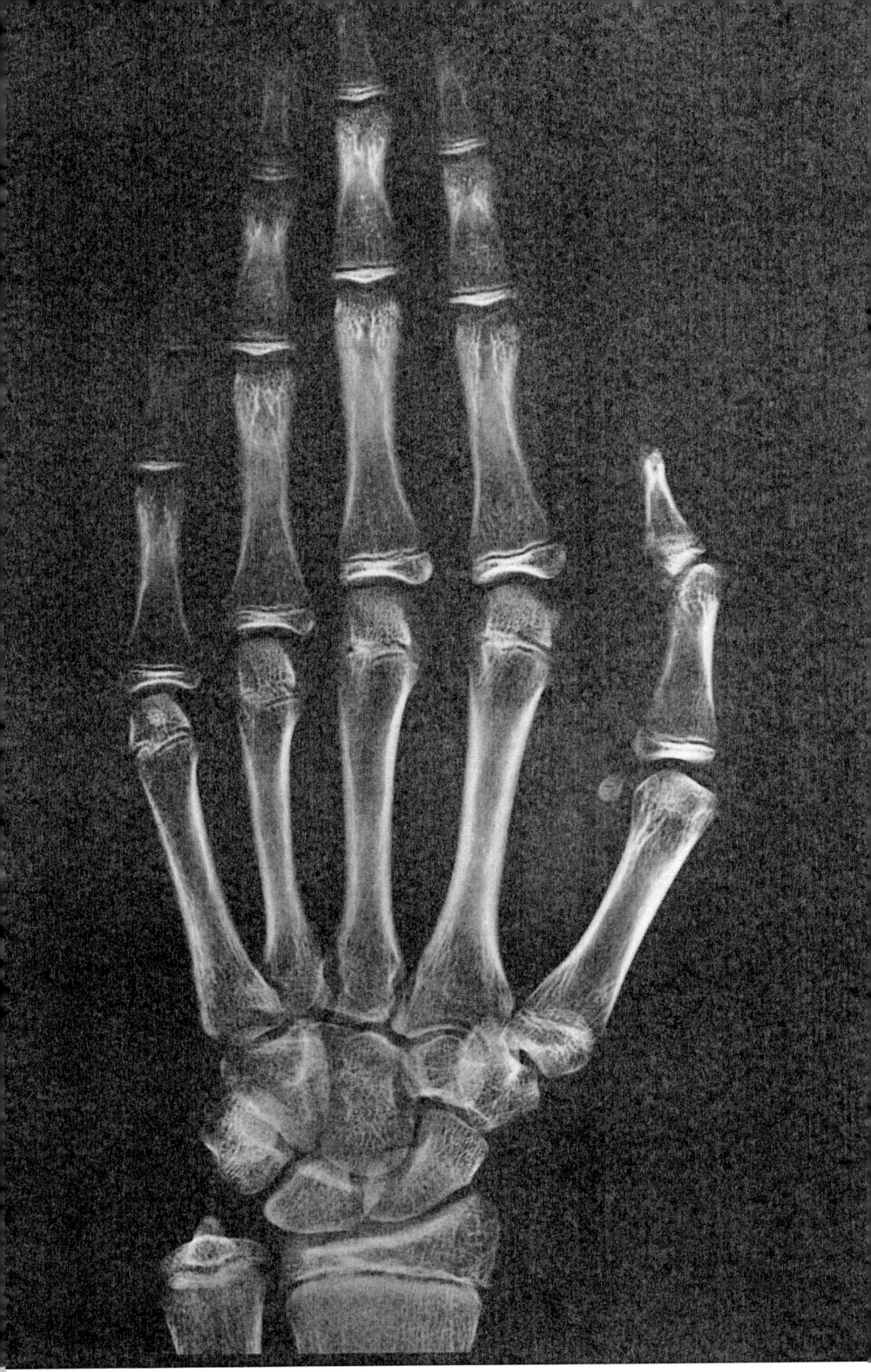

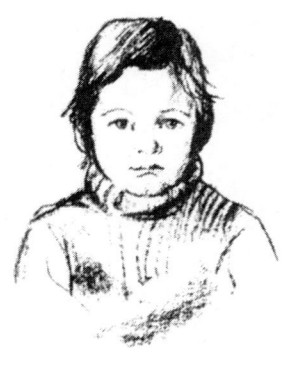

♂ 16 years

Radius and ulna: No changes.
Carpal bones: No changes.
Metacarpal bones: The epiphyses of the second, third, fourth, and fifth metacarpals have begun to fuse with their shafts.
Phalanges: Epiphysial- diaphysial fusion is well advanced in all the phalanges.

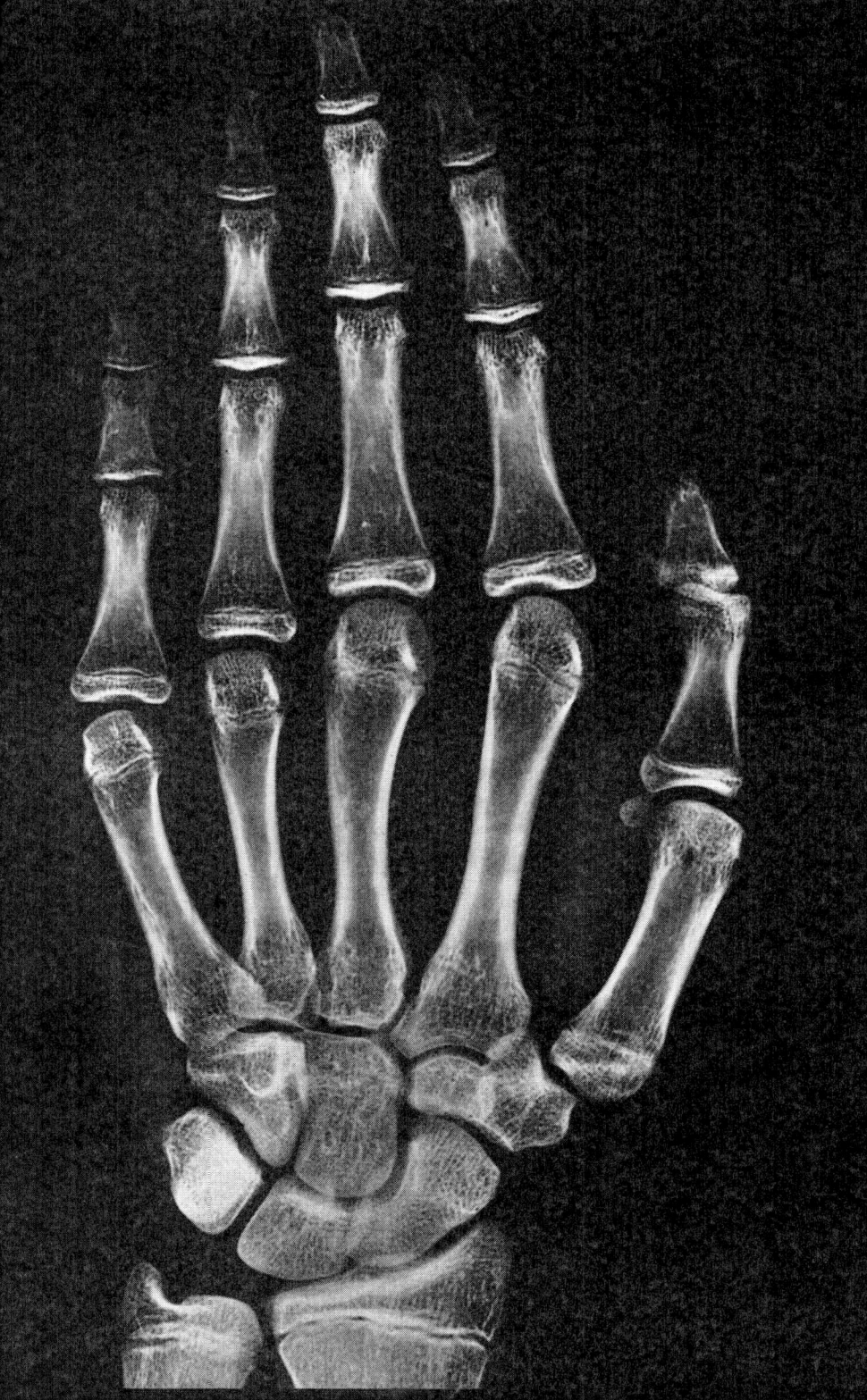

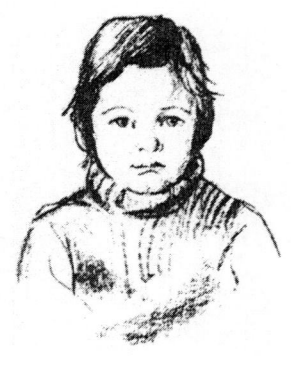

♂ 17 years

Radius and ulna: The thickness of the growth cartilage of the radius has become reduced preparatory to epiphysial-diaphysial fusion. Fusion has already begun in the ulna.

Metacarpal bones: The epiphyses of the metacarpals have recently fused with their shafts.

Phalanges: With the completion of fusion in the middle phalanges of the second, third and fourth fingers, all of the phalangeal epiphyses have fused with their shafts.

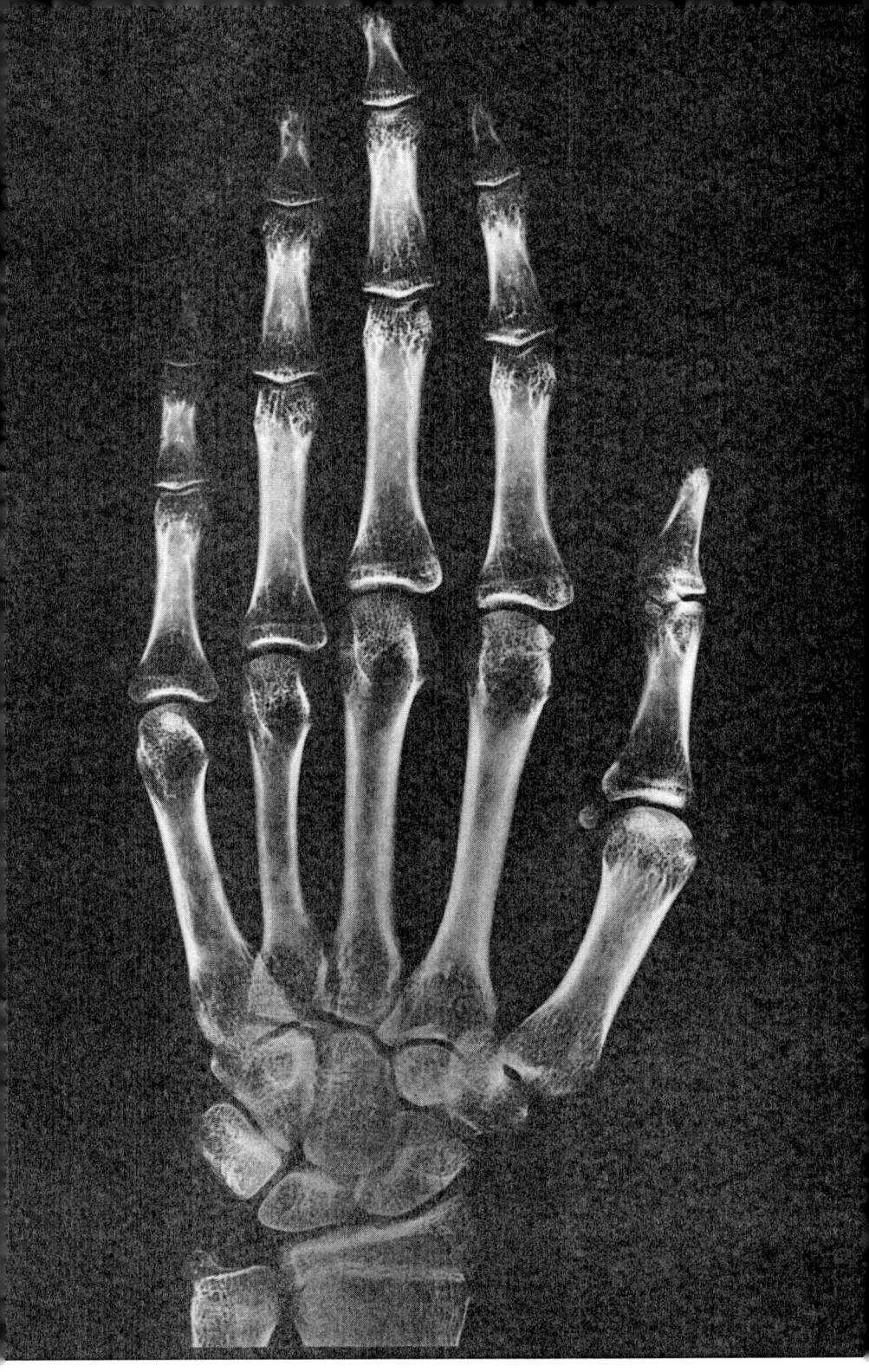

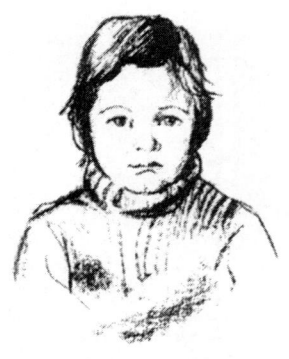

♂ 18 years

The fusion of the radial epiphysis with its shaft completes the skeletal maturation of the hand and wrist.

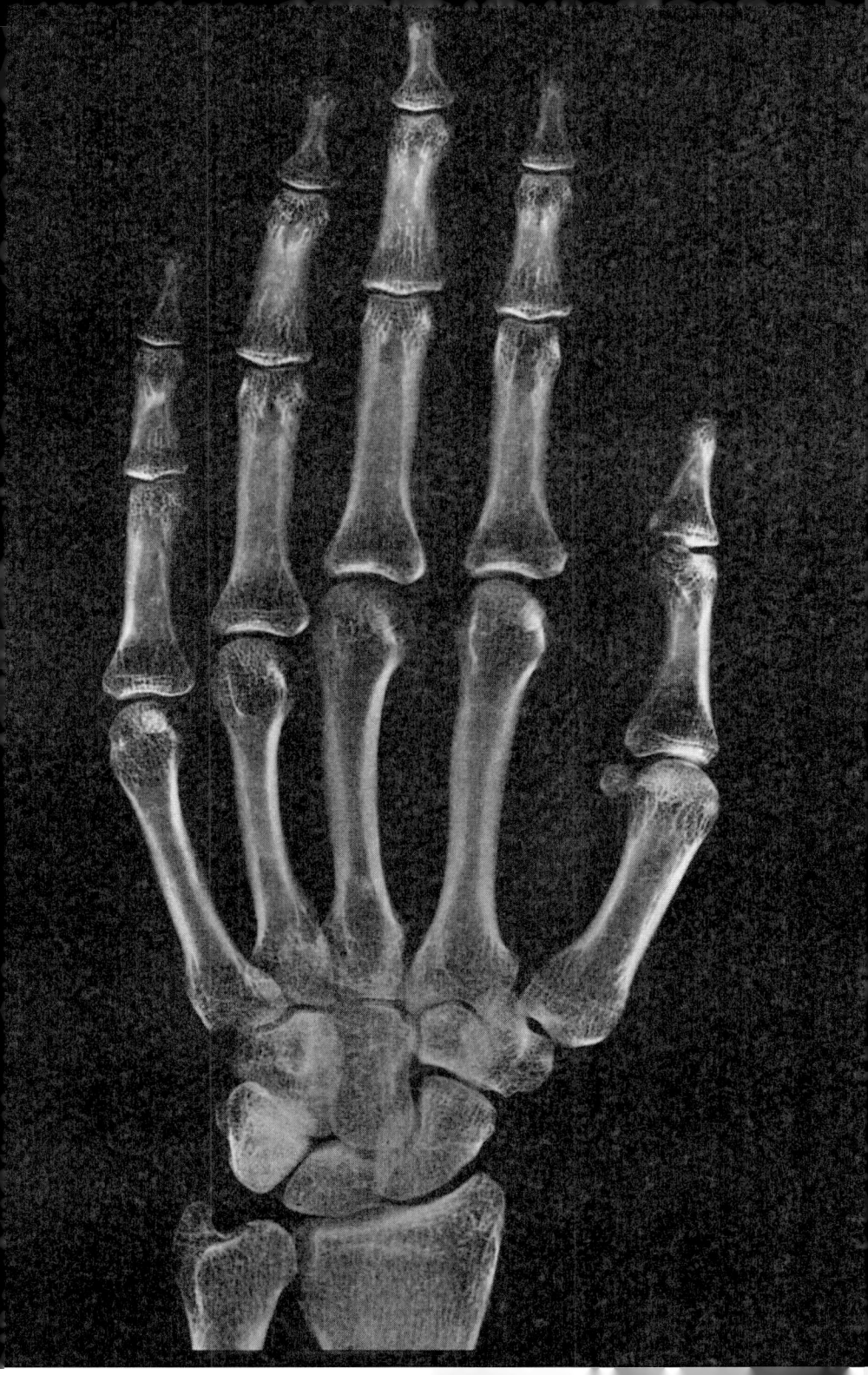

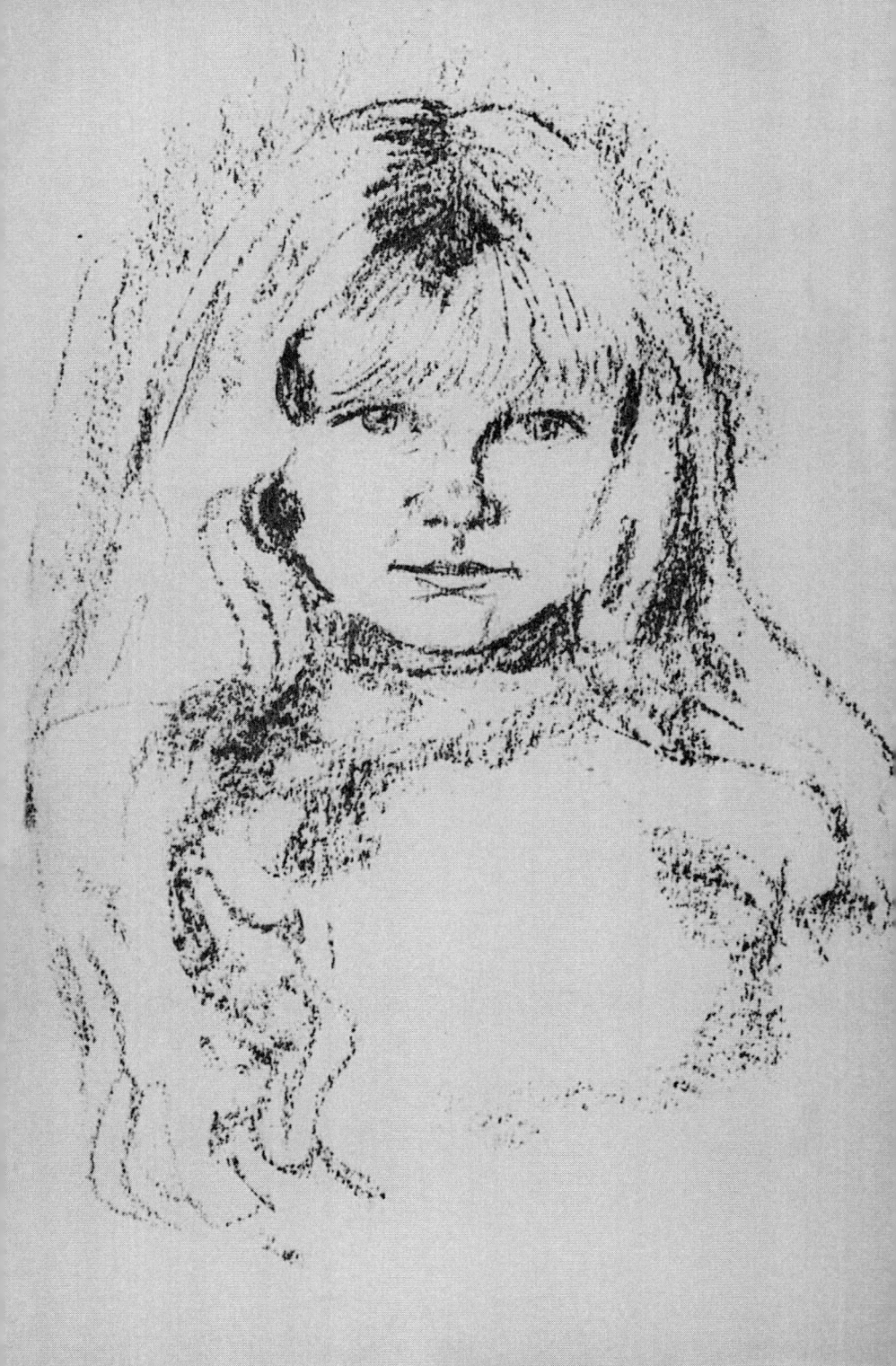

SKELETAL AGE OF GIRLS

Newborn
3 months
6 months
9 months
1 year
1 year and 3 months
1 year and 6 months
1 year and 9 months
2 years
2 years and 6 months
3 years
3 years and 6 months
4 years
5 years
6 years
7 years
8 years
9 years
10 years
11 years
12 years
13 years
14 years
15 years
16 years
17 years
18 years

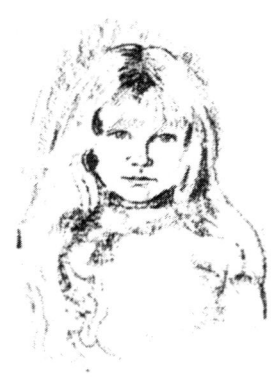

♀ Newborn

Radius and ulna: The distal ends are flared and the margins are somewhat flattened.
No ossification centers visible.
Carpal bones: No ossification centers visible.
Metacarpal bones: The shafts of the second to fifth metacarpals are slightly constricted in their middle portions. The proximal ends of the metacarpals are somewhat closer together than their distal ends and, consequently, the shafts appear to radiate out from the carpal area. No ossification centers visible.
Phalanges: The distal ends of the proximal and middle phalanges are rounded and their proximal ends are wider and flat. No ossification centers visible.

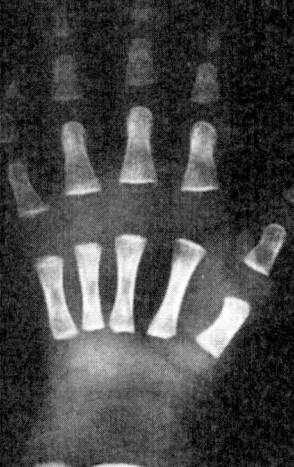

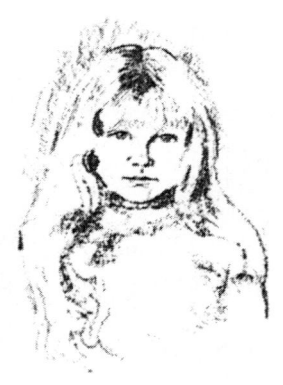

♀ 3 months

Radius and ulna: The beaklike projection on the radial side of the distal end of the ulna usually persist for several years. No ossification centers visible.

Carpal bones: A center of the ossification is now visible in both the capitate and the hamate. The capitate usually reaches this stage of development slightly earlier than the hamate.

Metacarpal bones: The ends of the metacarpals have increased in width relatively more than has the central potion of their shafts. The proximal ends of the metacarpals II and V and the distal end of metacarpal I are now more rounded than they were at birth. The proximal or future epiphysial margin of metacarpal I is flattened. No ossification center visible.

Phalanges: The phalanges have increased relatively more in length. Their epiphysial ends are flat and their nonepiphysial ends are rounded.

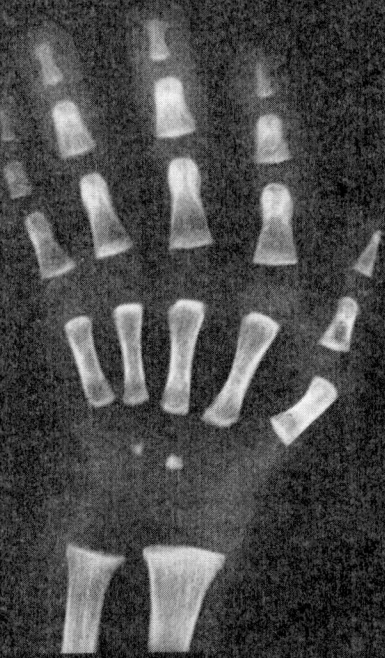

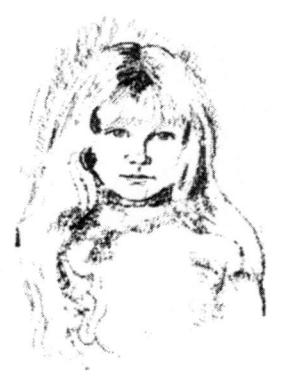

♀ 6 months

Radius and Ulna: No ossification centers visible.
Carpal bones: The hamate surface of the capitate is beginning to show flattening by a reduction in the degree of its convexity. The growth of the capitate and hamate center has brought them closer together.
Metacarpal bones: The bases of the third and fourth metacarpals are now distinctly rounded. No ossification centers visible.
Phalanges: No ossification centers visible.

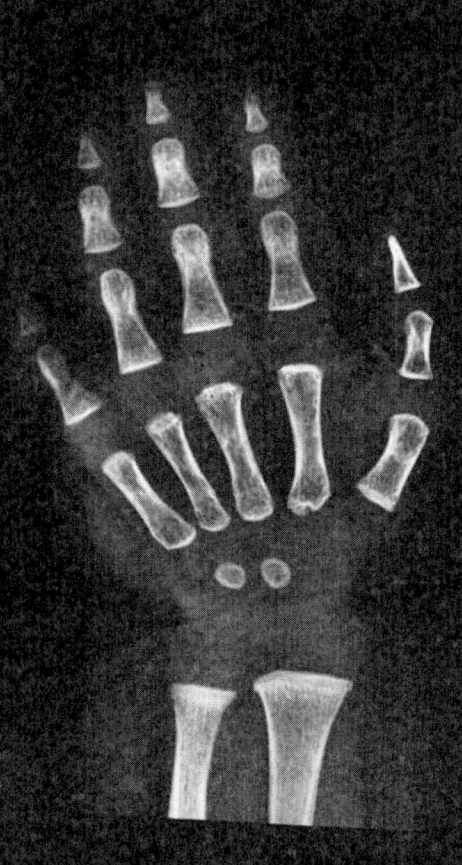

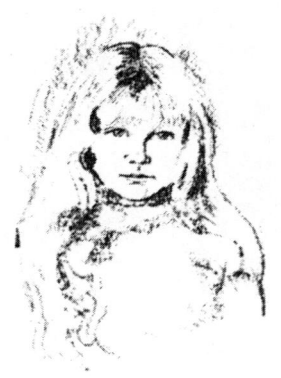

♀ 9 months

Radius and ulna: No ossification centers visible.
Carpal bones: The capitate is now larger and further advanced in its development than the hamate.
Metacarpal bones: No ossification centers visible.
Phalanges: No ossification centers visible.

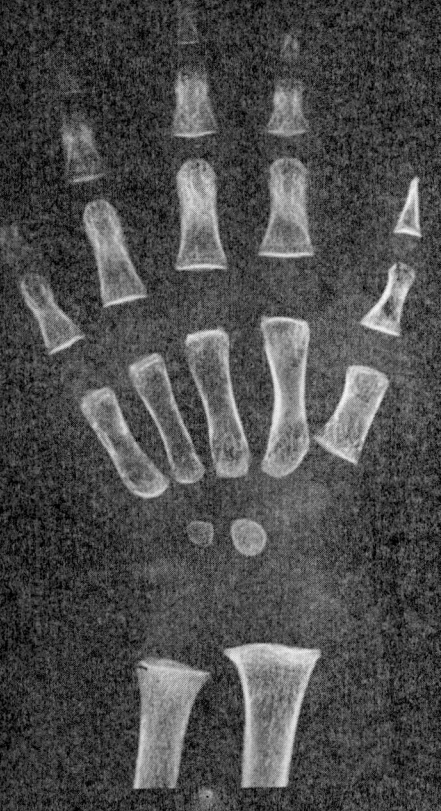

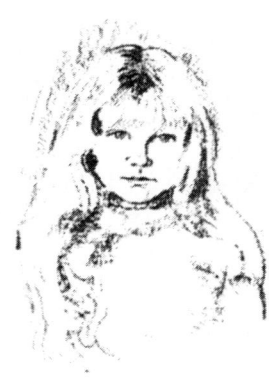

♀ 1 year

Radius and ulna: A flattened oval ossification center is now present in the distal epiphysis of the radius.
Carpal bones: No changes.
Metacarpal bones: The base of the second metacarpal has begun to enlarge. Ossification centers are visible of the second and third metacarpal.
Phalanges: Ossification center of the proximal phalanx of the second, third and fourth finger is just visible.

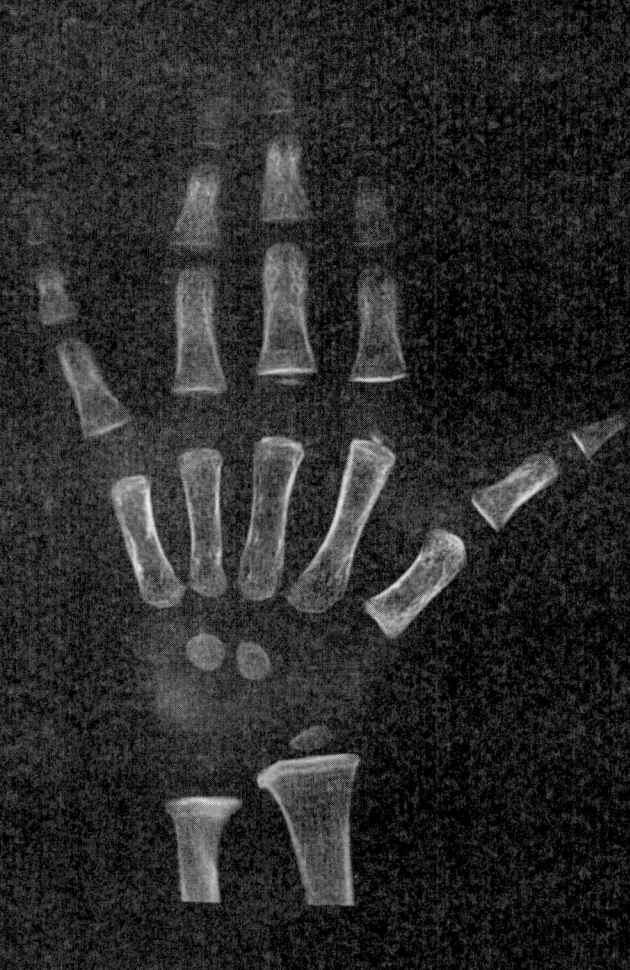

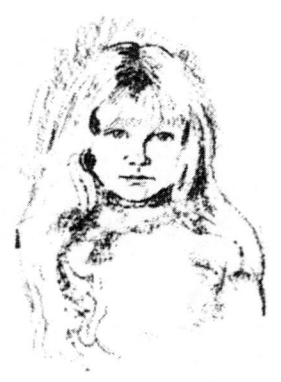

♀ 1 year and 3 months

Radius and ulna: Some growth of the ossification center of the radius
Carpol bones: The hamate is now somewhat wedge-shaped, its
proximal end being narrower than its distal end.
Metacarpal bones: Ossification has begun in the epiphysis of the
fourth metacarpal.
Phalanges: Ossification in the epiphysis of the distal phalanx of the
thumb has recently begun. Ossification of the proximal phalanx of
the fifth finger is just visible (due to the superior technique).

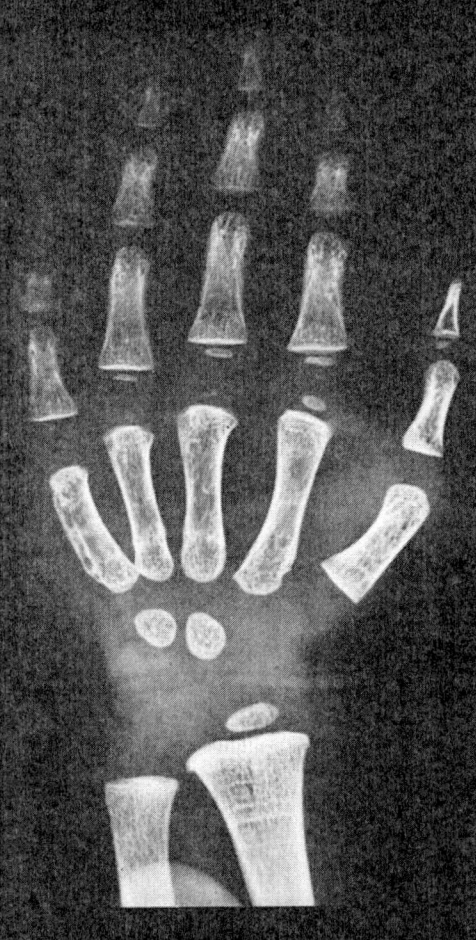

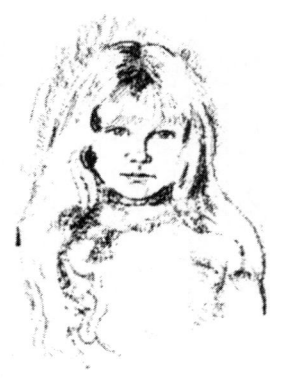

♀ 1 year and 6 months

Radius and ulna: No changes.

Carpal bones: The capitate and hamate have advanced in development.

Metacarpal bones: Ossification center of the epiphysis of the fifth metacarpal is now visible.

Phalanges: The epiphysis of the proximal phalanges of the second, third, fourth and fifth fingers are disc-shaped and their margins are fairly smooth.

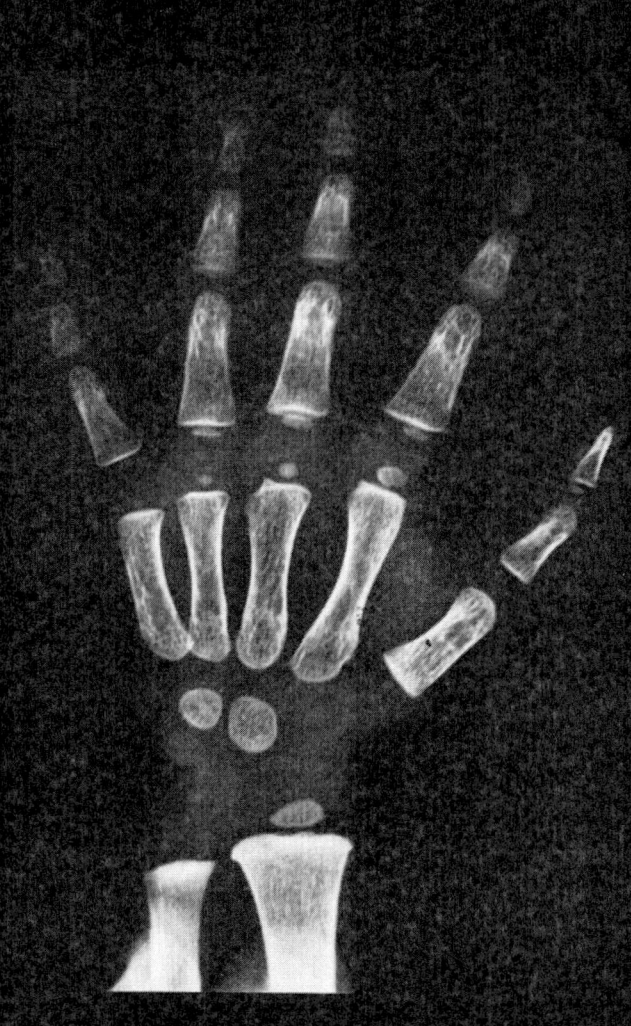

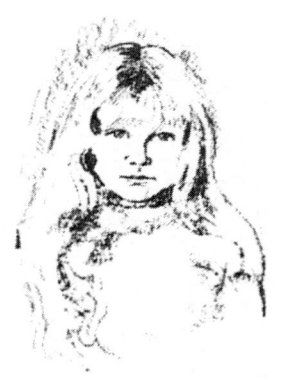

♀ 1 year and 9 months

Radius and ulna: No changes.
Carpal Bones: No changes.
Metacarpal Bones: A beginning of the ossification of the epiphyse of the first metacarpal becomes visible.
Phalanges: Ossification has begun in the epiphyses of the middle phalanx of the second, third, fourth and fifth finger and distal phalanx of the third and fourth finger.

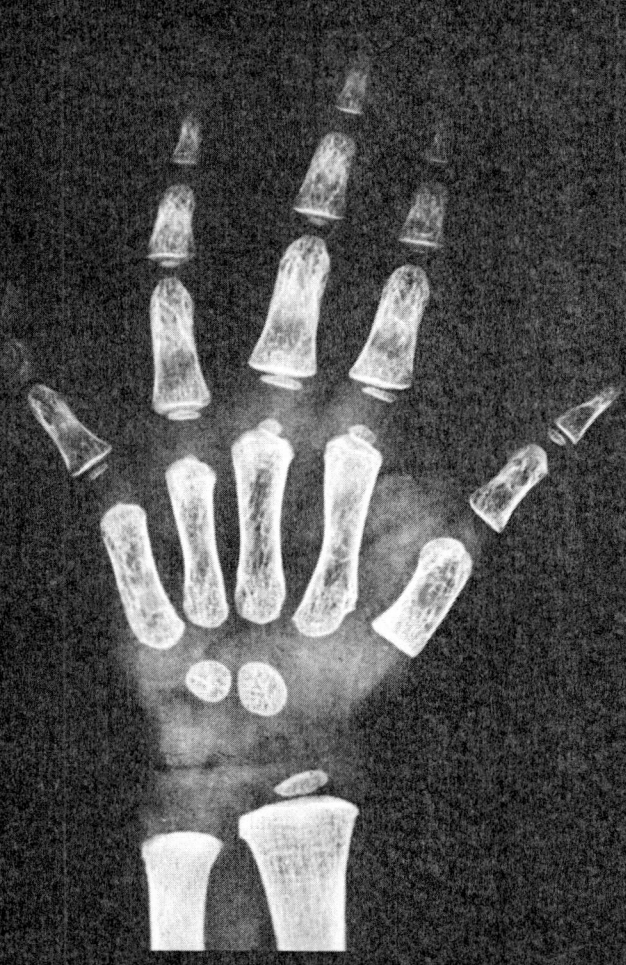

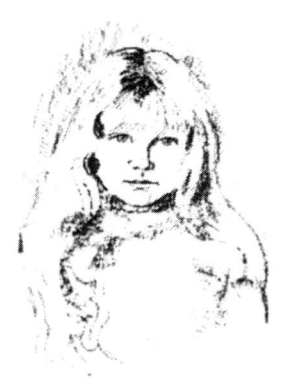

♀ **2 years**

Radius and ulna: The radial epiphysis now has a rounded lateral margin.

Carpal bones: The capitate surface of the hamate has flattened, and its proximal end is distincly narrower than its distal end. Its triquetral surface has begun to flatten. Ossification has begun in the triquetral.

Metacarpal bones: Ossification centers of the metacarpal bones have enlarged and more rounded.

Phalanges: Ossification has begun in the epiphysis of the proximal phalanx of the thumb. The epiphysis of the proximal phalanges of the second, third, fourth and fifth fingers are now more than half as wide as their shafts. Ossification of the epiphysis of the distal phalanges of the second and fifth finger become visible.

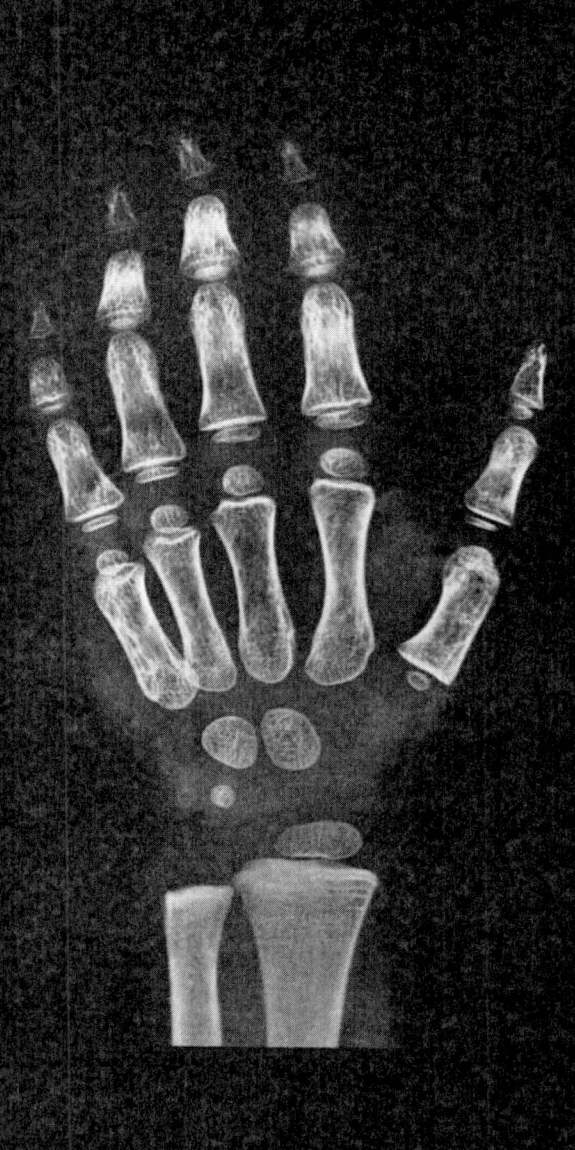

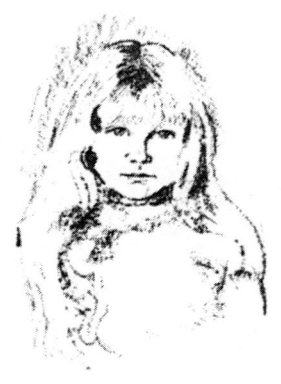

♀ 2 years and 6 months

Radius and ulna: The distal margins of the volar and dorsal surfaces of the radial epiphysis are now distinguishable. The distal volar margin can be seen as an oblique white line which lies proximal to the distal margin of the epiphysis and extends laterally from it ulnar tip.

Carpal bones: The carpal centers have enlarged and the triquetral center is more rounded.

Metacarpal bones: The proximal surfaces of the epiphysis of the third fourth and fifth metacarpals are now beginning to shape to their respective shafts.

Phalanges: Growth of the ossification centers which become more disc-shaped.

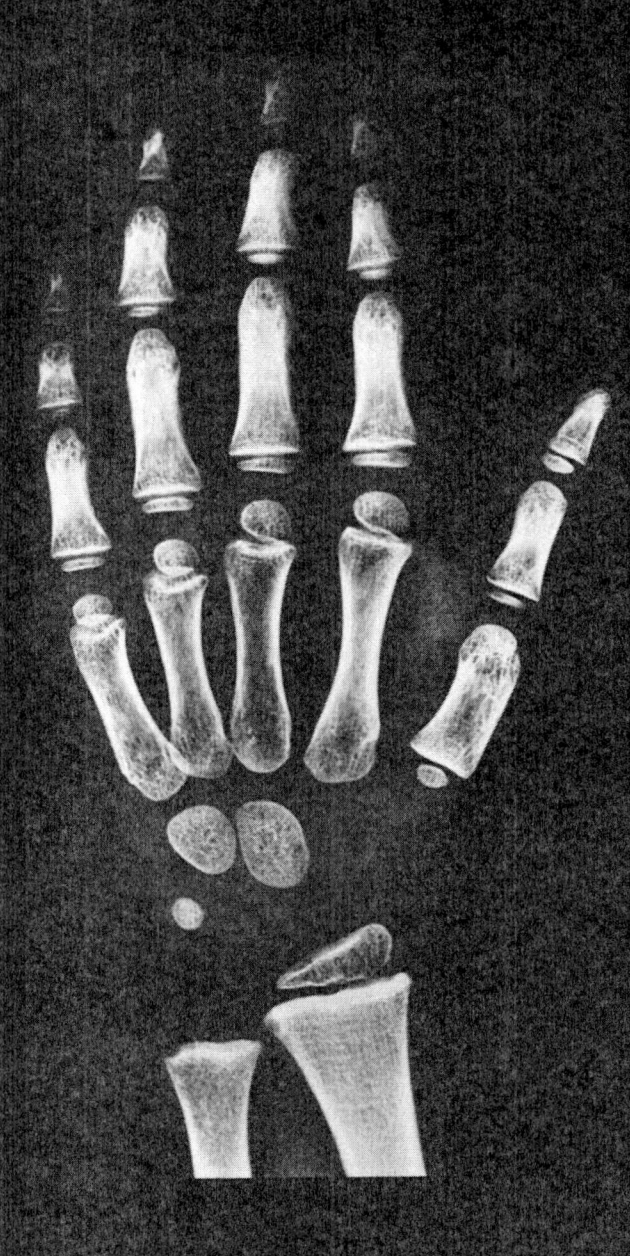

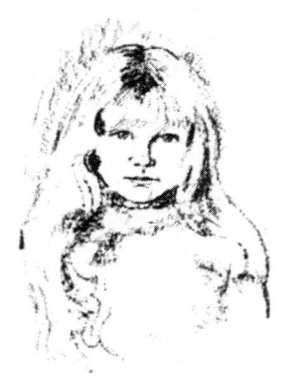

♀ 3 years

Radius and ulna: Some more flattening of the radius epiphyse.
Carpal Bones: The lunate center is now visible.
Metacarpal Bones: No changes.
Phalanges: No changes.

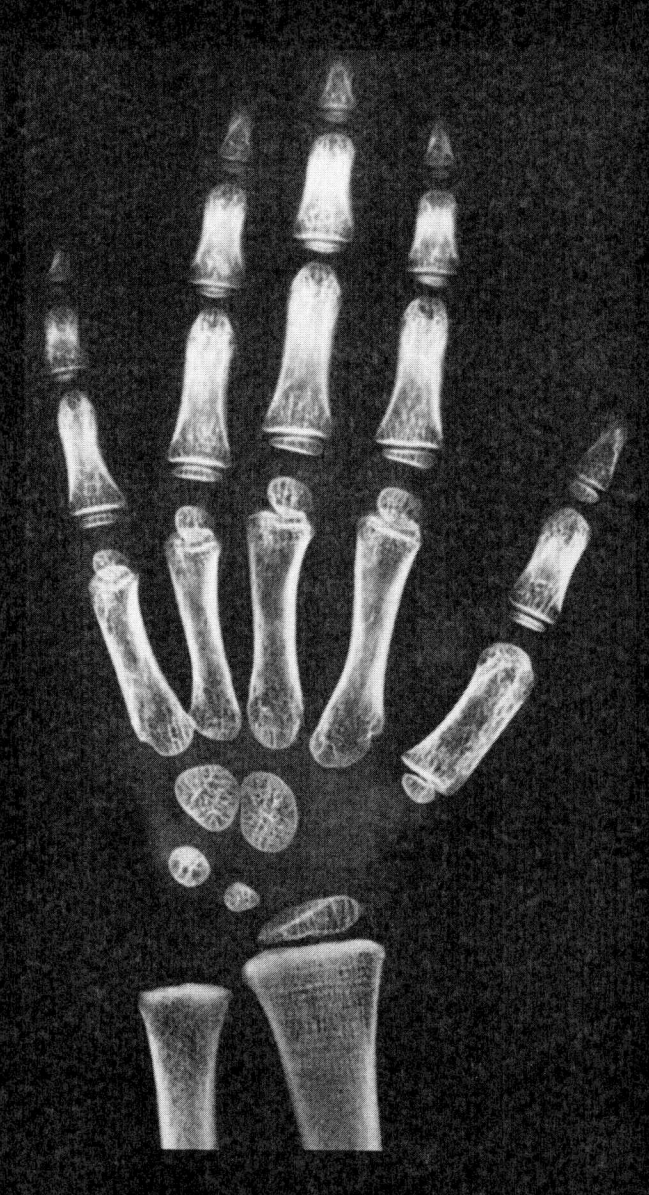

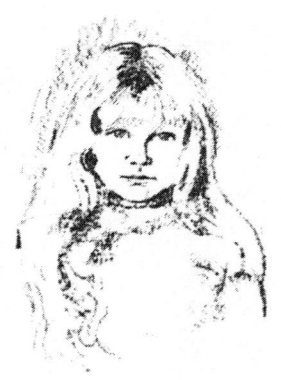

♀ 3 years and 6 months

Radius and ulna: No changes.
Carpal Bones: A center of ossification has appeared in the trapezium.
Metacarpal Bones: No changes.
Phalanges: No changes.

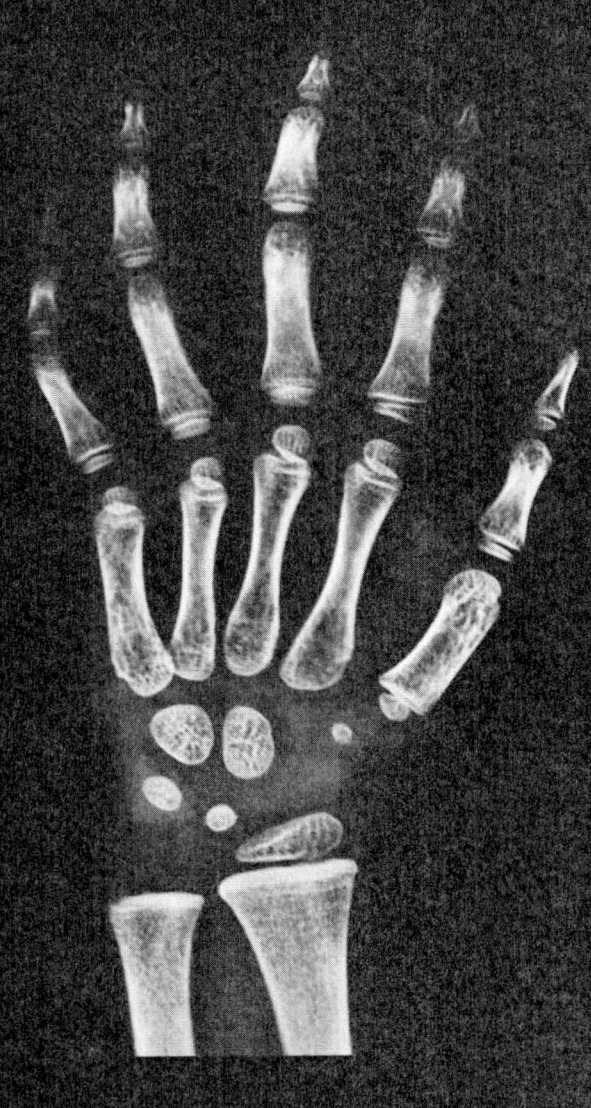

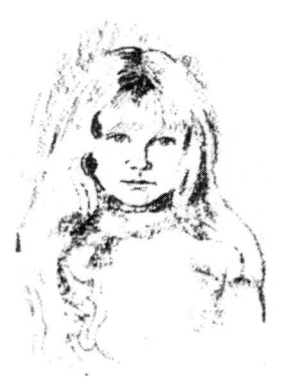

♀ 4 years

Radius and ulna: No changes.

Carpal Bones: Ossifications centres are now visible in the scaphoid and trapezoid.

Metacarpal Bones: The base of the second metacarpal become slighty concave.

Phalanges: The articular surfaces of the epiphyses of the proximal phalanx of the second and third finger have become slighty concave as the shape to the heads of the corresponding metacarpals.

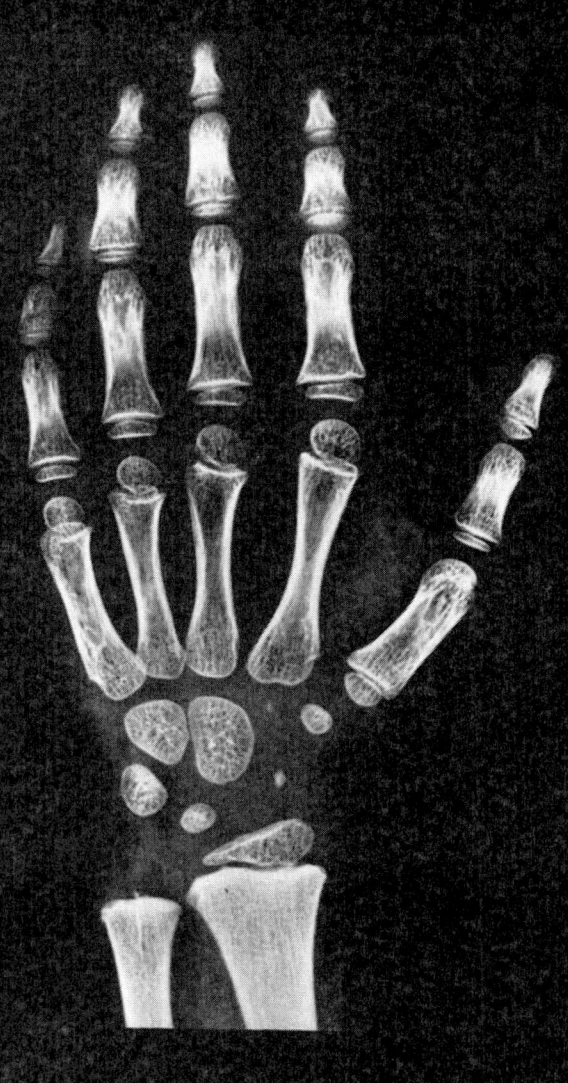

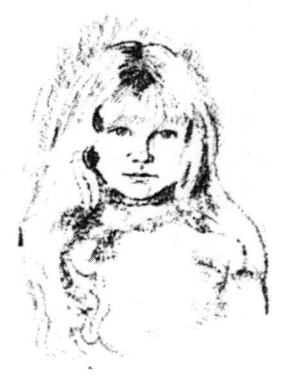

♀ 5 years

Radius and ulna: No changes.
Carpal bones: The dorsal and volar aspects of the capitate surface of the lunate are beginning to be distinguishable. The curved white linear marking near the distal margin represents a part of the volar surface. The center of the trapezoid is much enlarged and rounded. The surface of the trapezium which will later articulate with the first metacarpal has begun to flatten. The ossification center of the scaphoid has enlarged and become ovoïd.
Metacarpal bones: The base of the second metacarpal adjacent to the trapezoid is beginning to become slightly concave.
Phalanges: No changes.

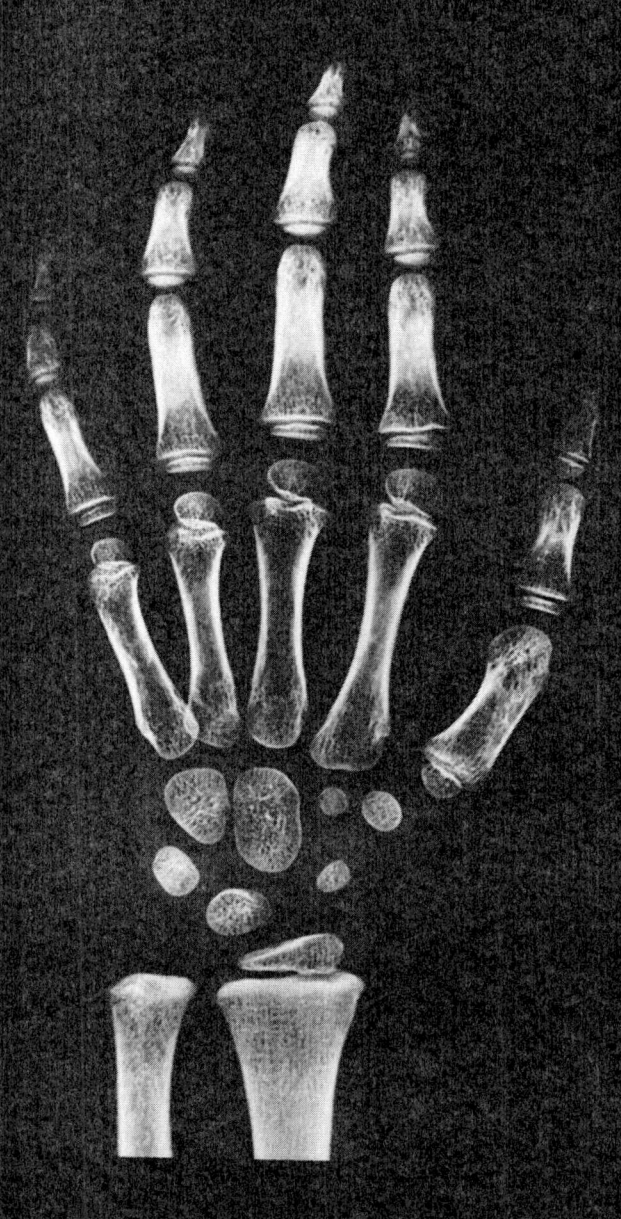

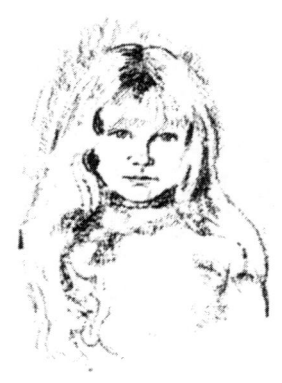

♀ 6 years

Radius and ulna: Enlargement of the radial epiphysis.
Carpal bones: The contiguous margins of the capitate and hamate now overlap. The space between the trapezoid and trapezium has become much reduced. An indentation is visible in the radial margin of the capitatum. The hamate surface of the triquetral has begun to flatten and its ulnar margin has become less convex.
Metacarpal bones: The concavity of the base of the second metacarpal is more prominent now.
Phalanges: The epiphysis of the distal phalanges are now as wide as their shafts.

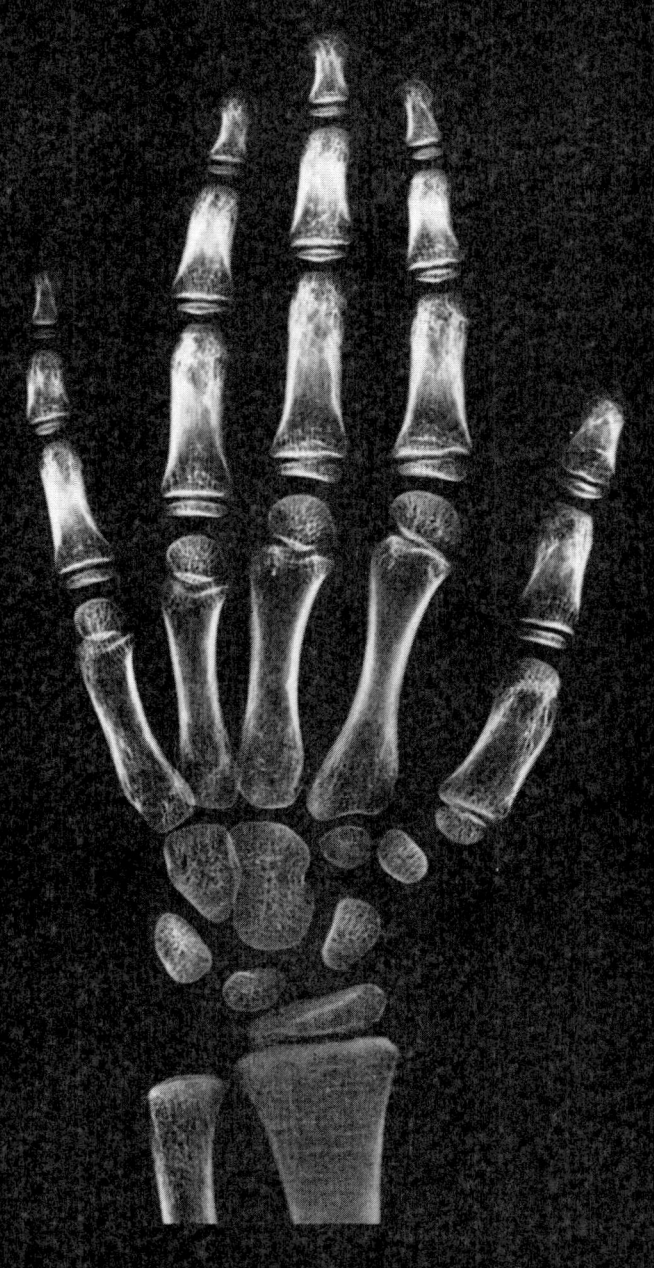

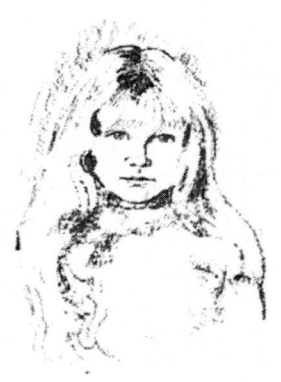

♀ 7 years

Radius and ulna: Modeling of the carpal articular surface of the radius has occured. An ossification center is now present in the distal epiphysis of the ulna.

Carpal bones: The capitate surface of the scaphoid is now slightly concave. The portion of the proximal margin of the trapezium which will later articulate with the scaphoid is now somewhat flattened. A similar flattening can be seen in the future capitate articular surface of the trapezoid. The spaces between the scaphoid, lunate, and capitate and between lunate and triquetral have been considerably reduced. The volar and dorsal margins of the trapezoid are now distinguishable.

Metacarpal bones: No changes.

Phalanges: The epiphysis of the proximal phalanges of the second, third, fourth and fifth finger is shaping to the contour of the epiphysis of the adjacent metacarpals.

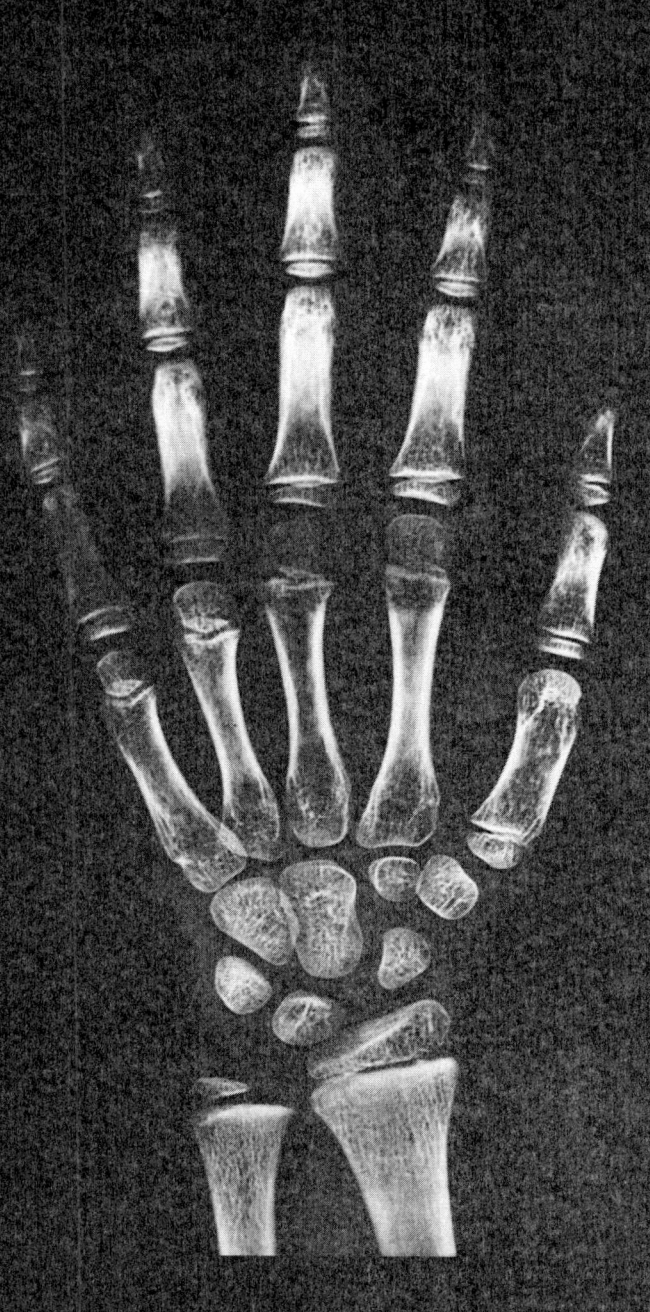

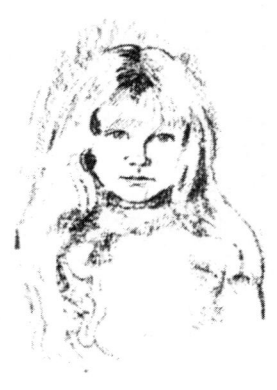

♀ 8 years

Radius and ulna: The ulnar epiphysis has increased in size, and its proximal margin has begun to shape to its shafts.

Carpal bones: The lunate surface of the triquetral is now flattened. The lunate has shaped further to the adjacent surfaces of the capitate and the radial epiphysis. The outline of the volar margin of the capitate surface of the scaphoïd is beginning to be discernible. The most medial part of the trapezium overlaps the lateral margin of the trapezoid. The scaphoïd surface of the trapezoïd has flattened. The metacarpal surfaces of the capitate are beginning to form.

Metacarpal bones: The capitate articular surface of the second metacarpal has begun to elongate.

Phalanges: The epiphysis of the distal phalanges of the second, third, fourth and fifth fingers are shaping to the trochlear surfaces of the middle phalanges.

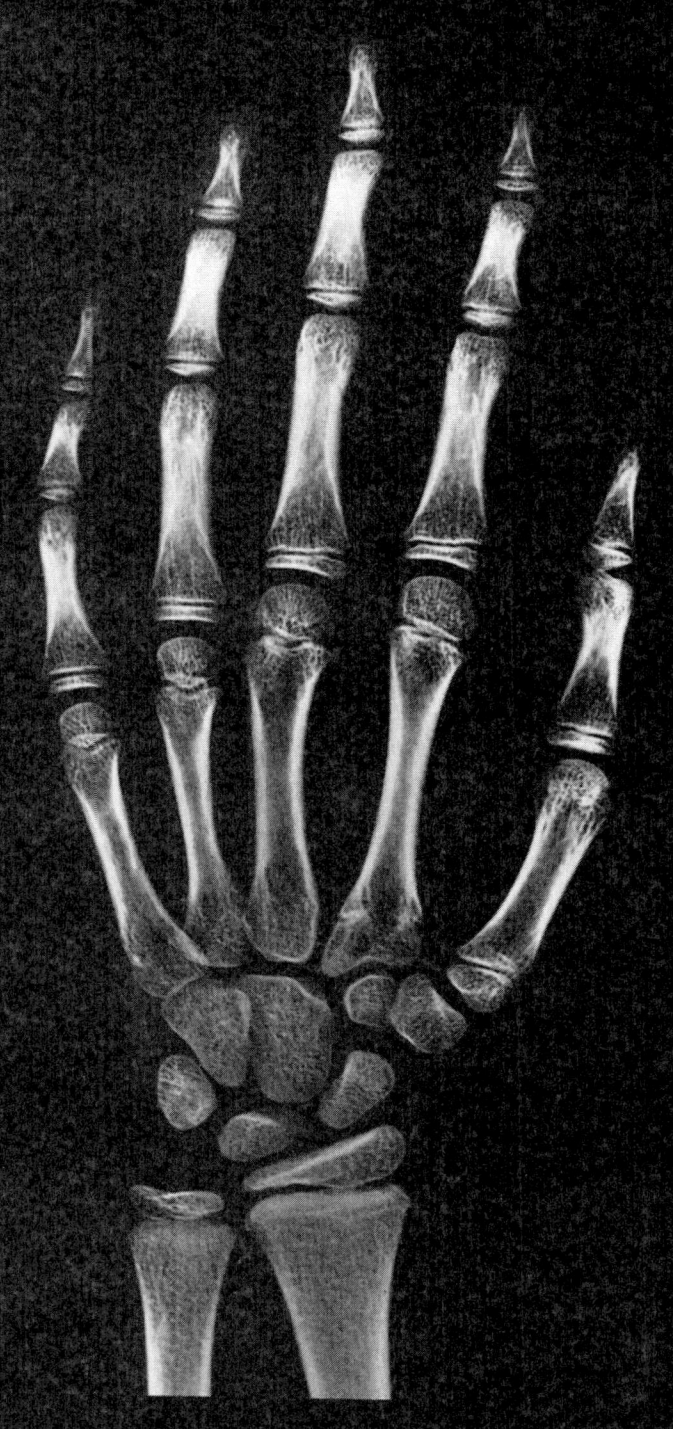

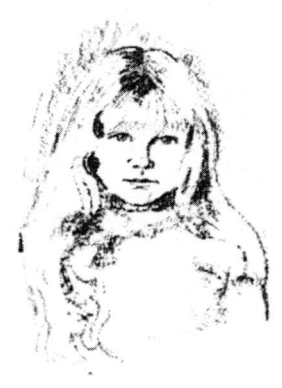

♀ 9 years

Radius and ulna: The ulnar epiphysis has now flattened and widened to form a bony plate. Its distal margin is concave and there is a distinct styloid process.

Carpal bones: The volar and dorsal margins of the hamate can now be distinguished. The scaphoid and radial surfaces of the lunate are beginning to defined. Much of the volar and dorsal surfaces of the trapezoid are now distinguishable. The rather advanced ossification center of the pisiform can be seen volar to the triquetral.

Metacarpal bones: The proximal surfaces of the epiphysis of the second, third, fourth and fifth metacarpals are shaping further to the ends of their shafts. Parts of the volar margins of these epiphysis are now visible.

Phalanges: The epiphysis of the proximal middle phalanges of the second, third and fourth fingers are now as wide as their shafts.

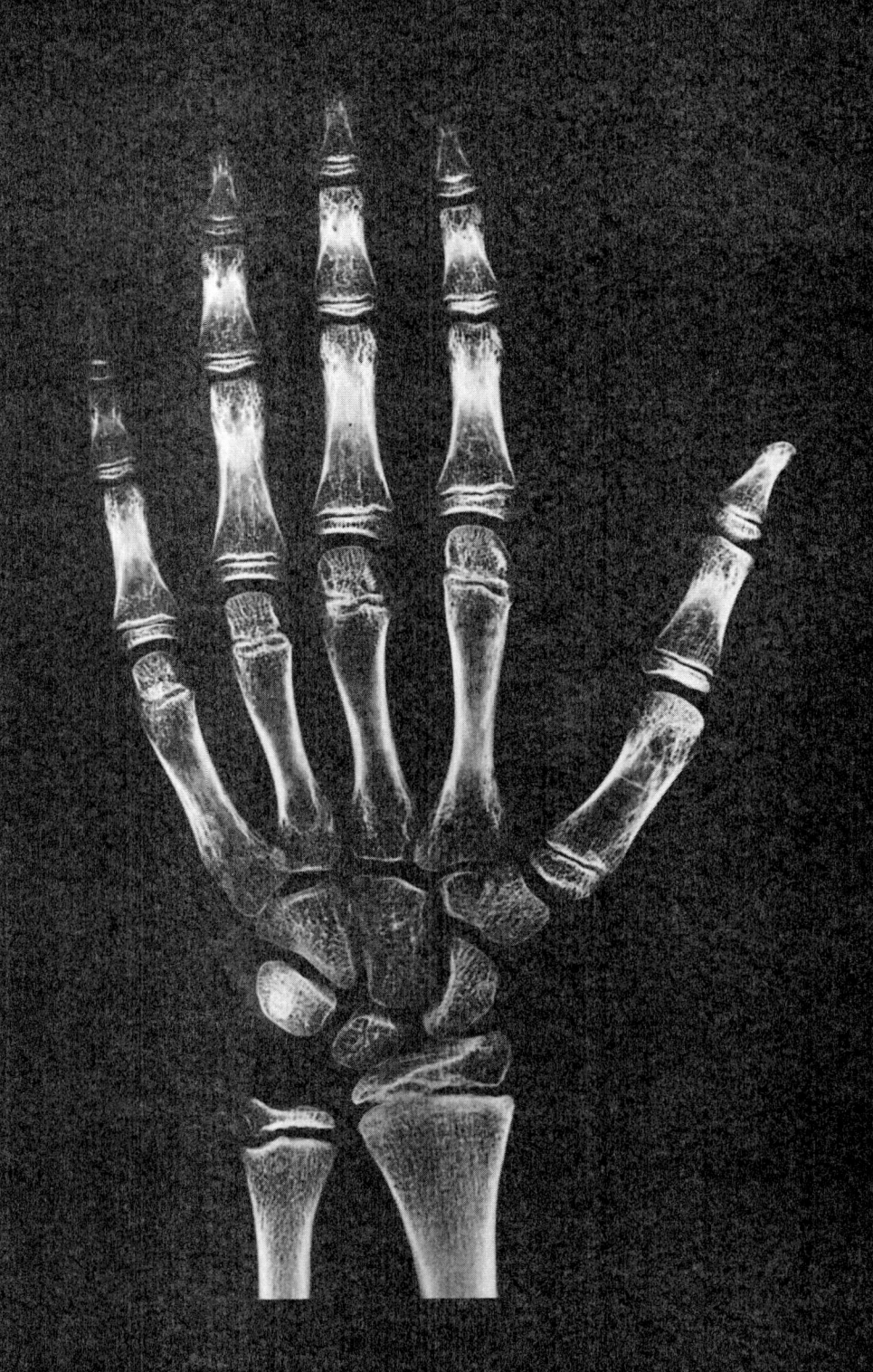

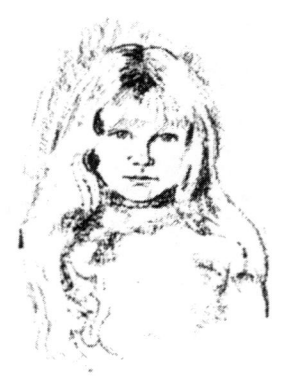

♀ 10 years

Radius and ulna: No changes.

Carpal bones: The outline of the tip of the hamulus of the hamate is now discernible. The pisiform has enlarged.

Metacarpal bones: An indentitation has developed in the articular surface of the epifysis of the first metacarpal.

Phalanges: The developing trochlear surfaces on the distal ends of the proximal phalanges of the second, third and fourth fingers now have shallow central indentations.

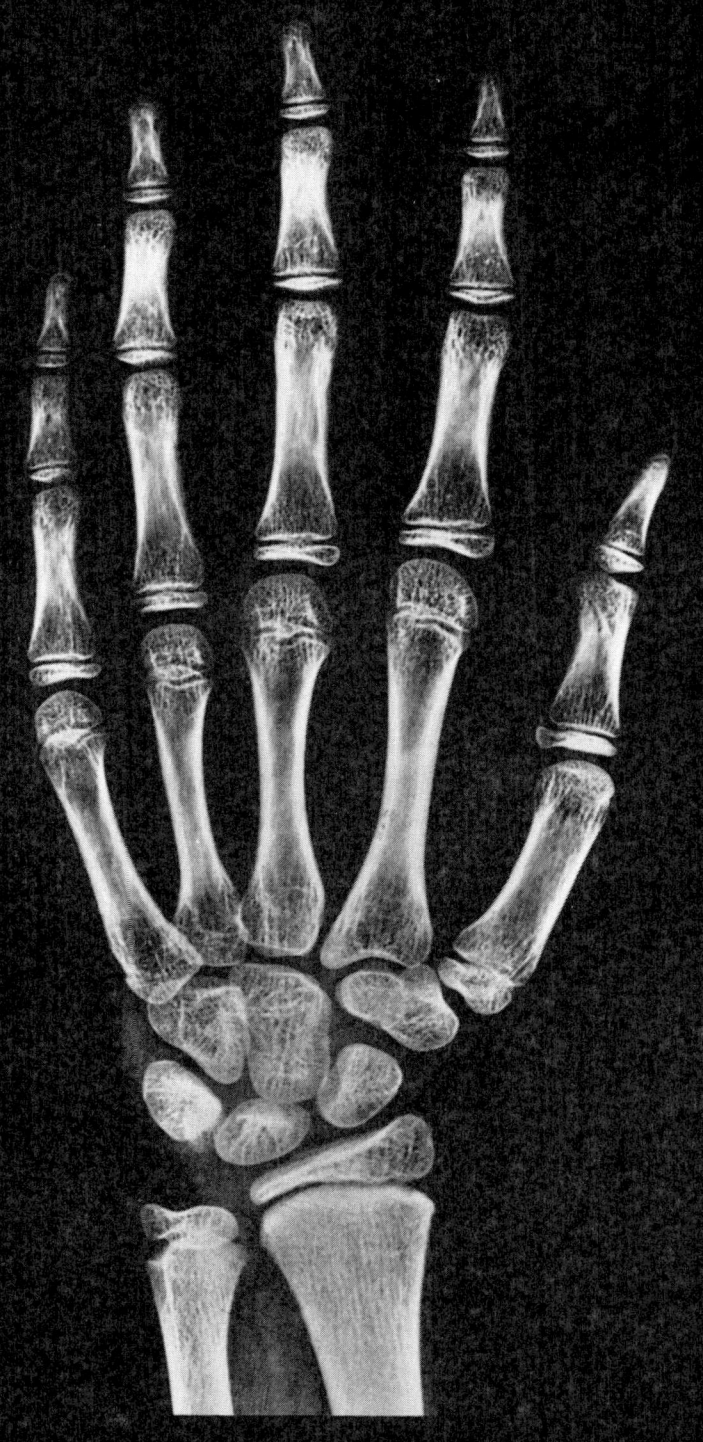

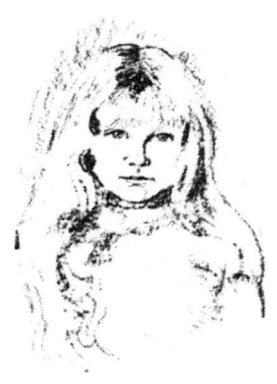

♀ 11 years

Radius and ulna: The proximal margin of the radial epiphysis has
adjusted further to the shape of the distal end of its shafts. The ulnar
epiphysis is shaping to the adjacent surface of the radius and to the
radial portion of the end of its own shaft.
Carpal bones: The hook of the hamulus appears as a triangular
outline within the shadow of the hamate. Further reciprocal shaping
has occured in the adjacent surfaces of the capitate and scaphoid. The
medial half of the trapezium now projects distally toward the base of
the second metacarpal, with which it will later articulate.
Metacarpal bones: the base of the second metacarpal has shaped
further to the adjacent surface of the trapezoid. The ossification
center of the sesamoïd in the tendon of the adductor pollicis is now
visible, just medial to the head of the first metacarpal.
Phalanges: All the epiphyses of the phalanges now cap their shafts.

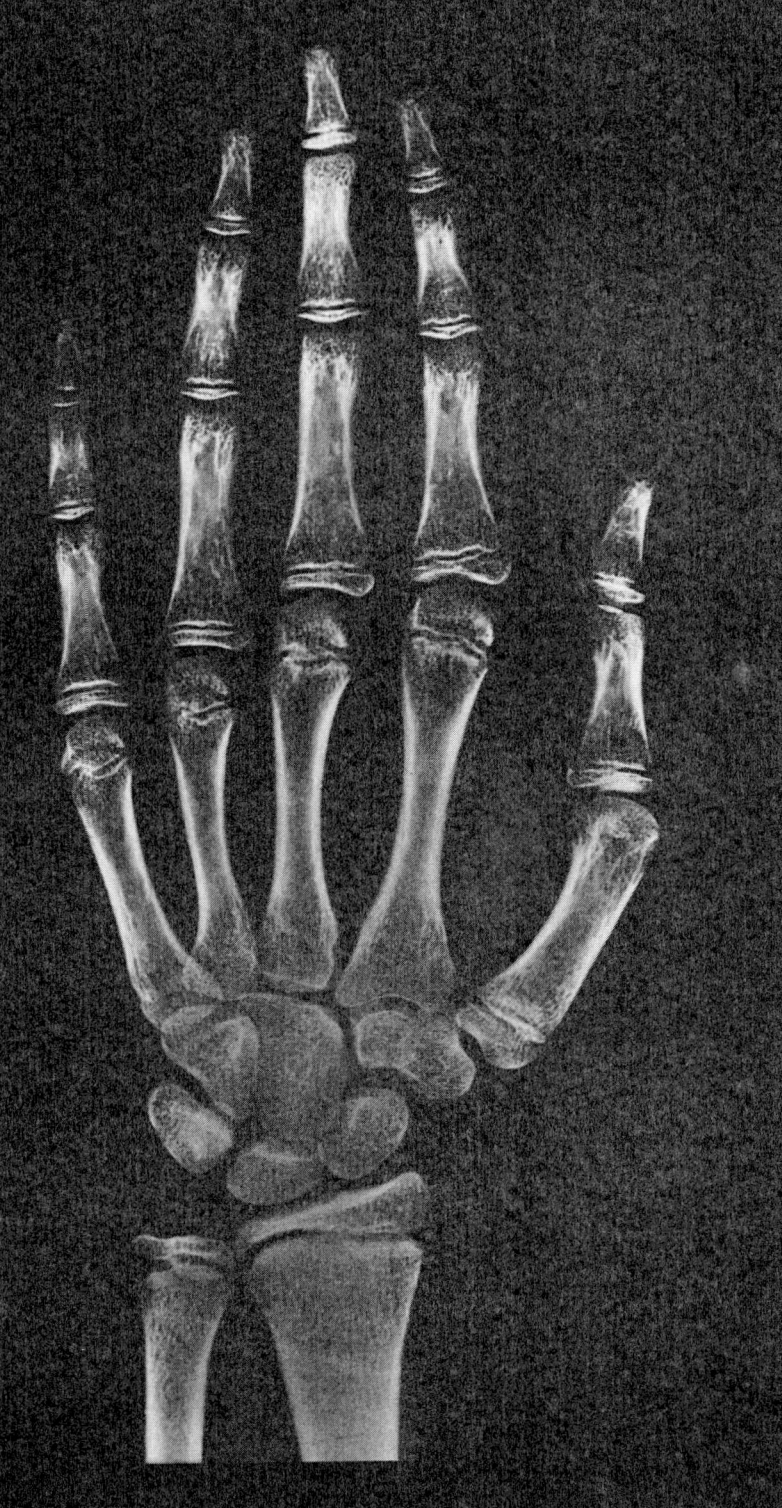

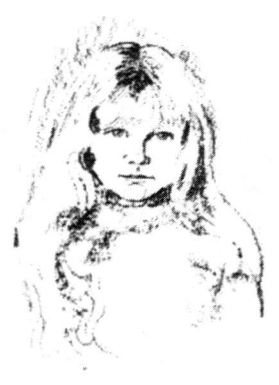

♀ 12 years

Radius and ulna: The radial epiphysis caps its shaft and its ulnar articular surface has flattened. The epiphysis of the ulna has shaped further to the distal end of its shaft and it's styloid process has become more prominent.

Carpal bones: The various articular surfaces of the capitate, hamate, trapezoid and trapezium are now well defined. This marking, which outlines the developing tubercle of the scaphoid, has become more distinct. The definitive shape of the joint between the scaphoid, trapezoid and trapezium is now established. The proximal borders of its dorsal and volar surfaces are now distinguishable.

Metacarpal bones: Growth of the sesamoid.

Phalanges: The radiolucent spaces between the various epiphyses and their shafts represent the epiphysial cartilage plates, all of which are now as thin as they will become until epiphysial-diaphysial fusion begins.

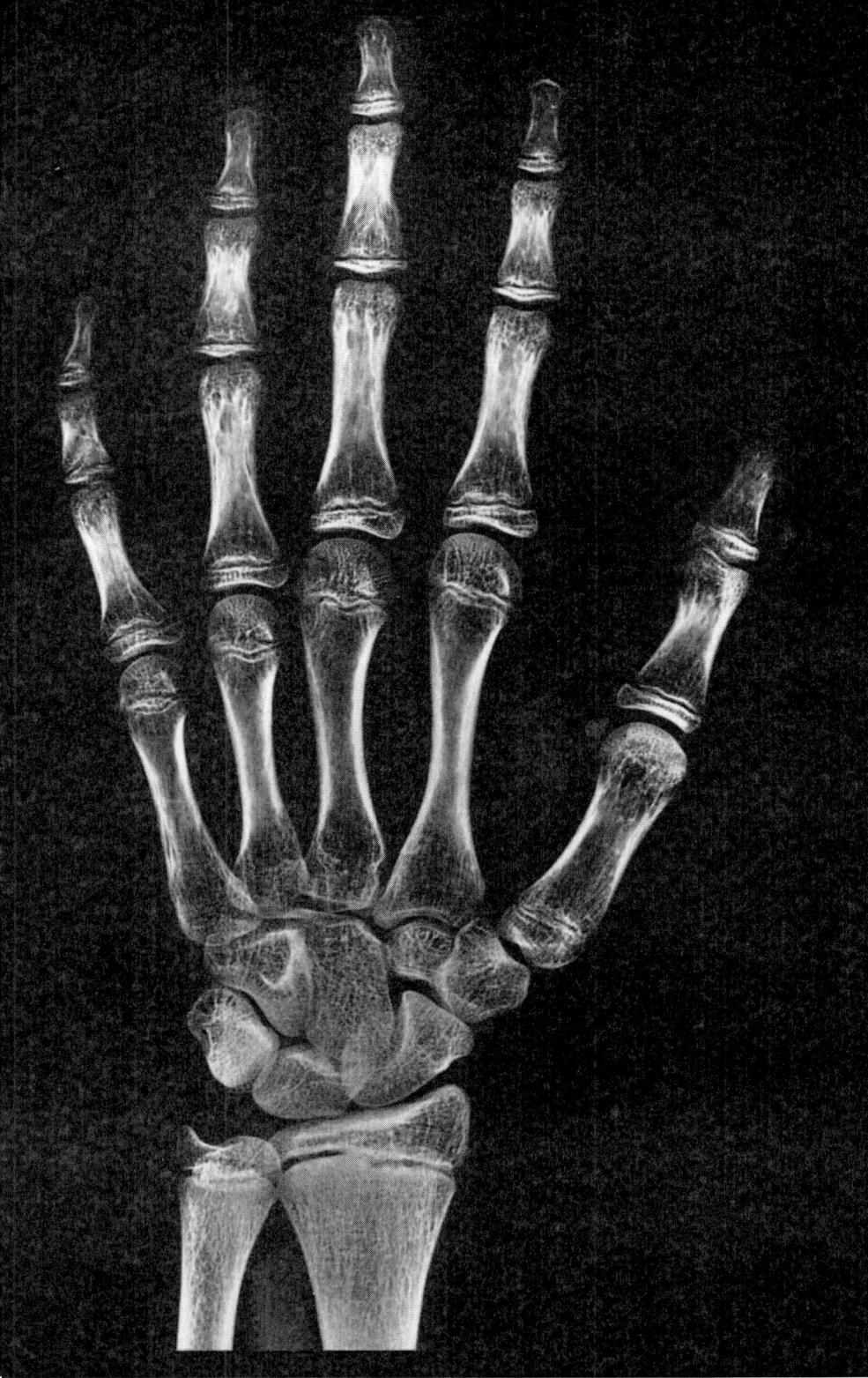

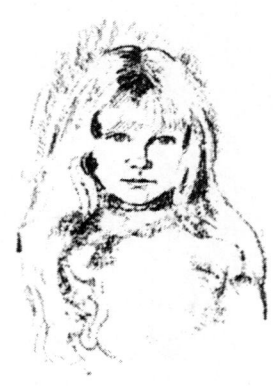

♀ 13 years

Radius and ulna: No changes.
Carpal bones: The form of all the carpals is now essentially adult.
Metacarpals bones: No changes.
Phalanges: The epiphyses of the distal phalanx of the thumb has begun to fuse with its shaft.
There are more accessory sesamoid bones present.

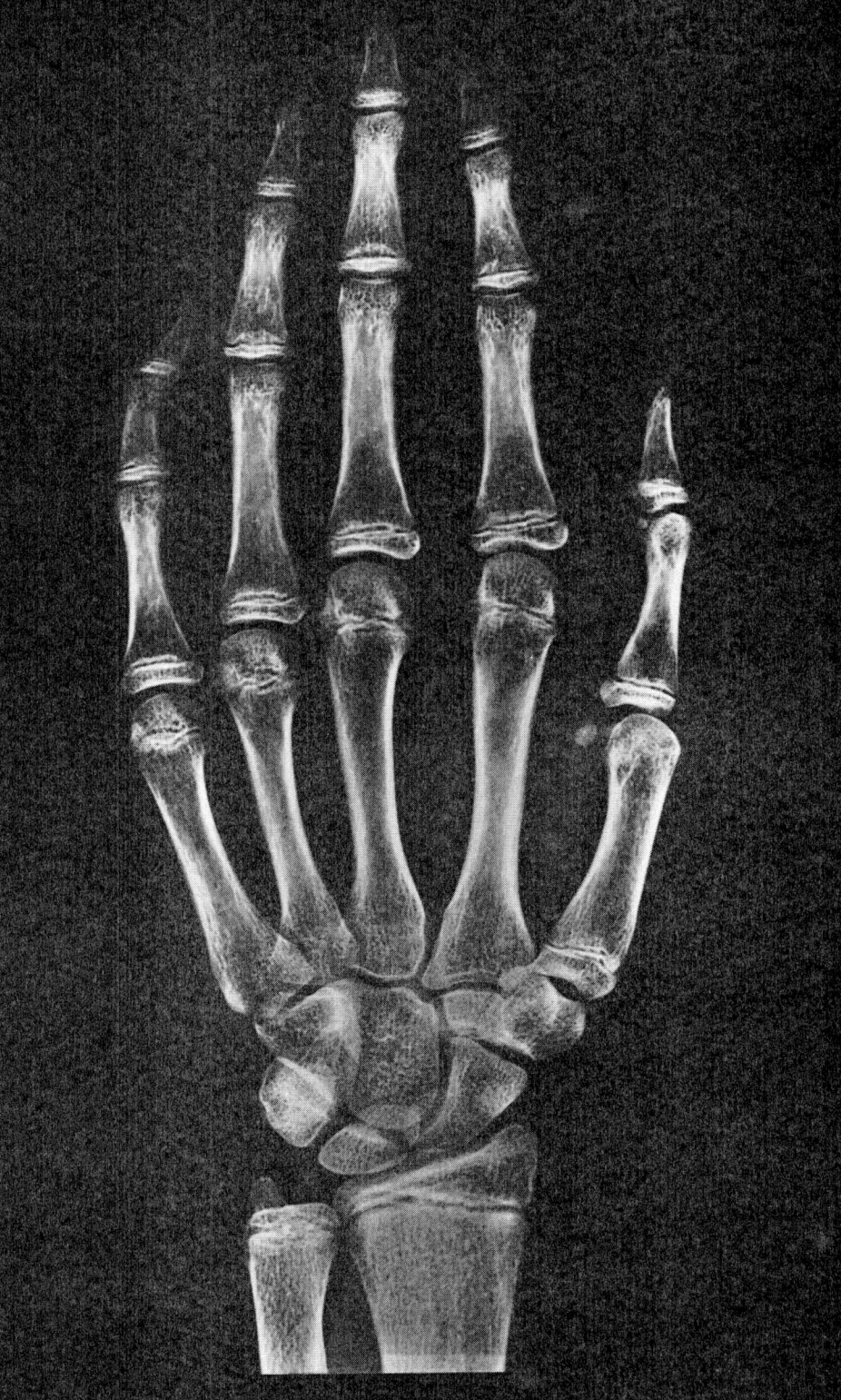

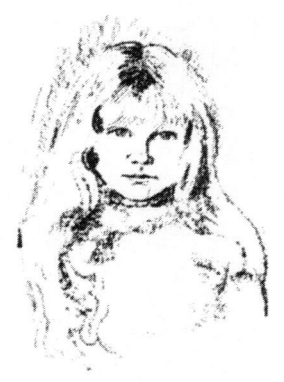

♀ 14 years

Radius and ulna: The epiphysial cartilage plates of the radius and ulna are now appreciably reduced in thickness.

Carpal bones: No changes.

Metacarpal bones: Epiphysial-diaphysial fusion began in the first metacarpal.

Phalanges: The epiphyses of the distal phalanges are fused now.

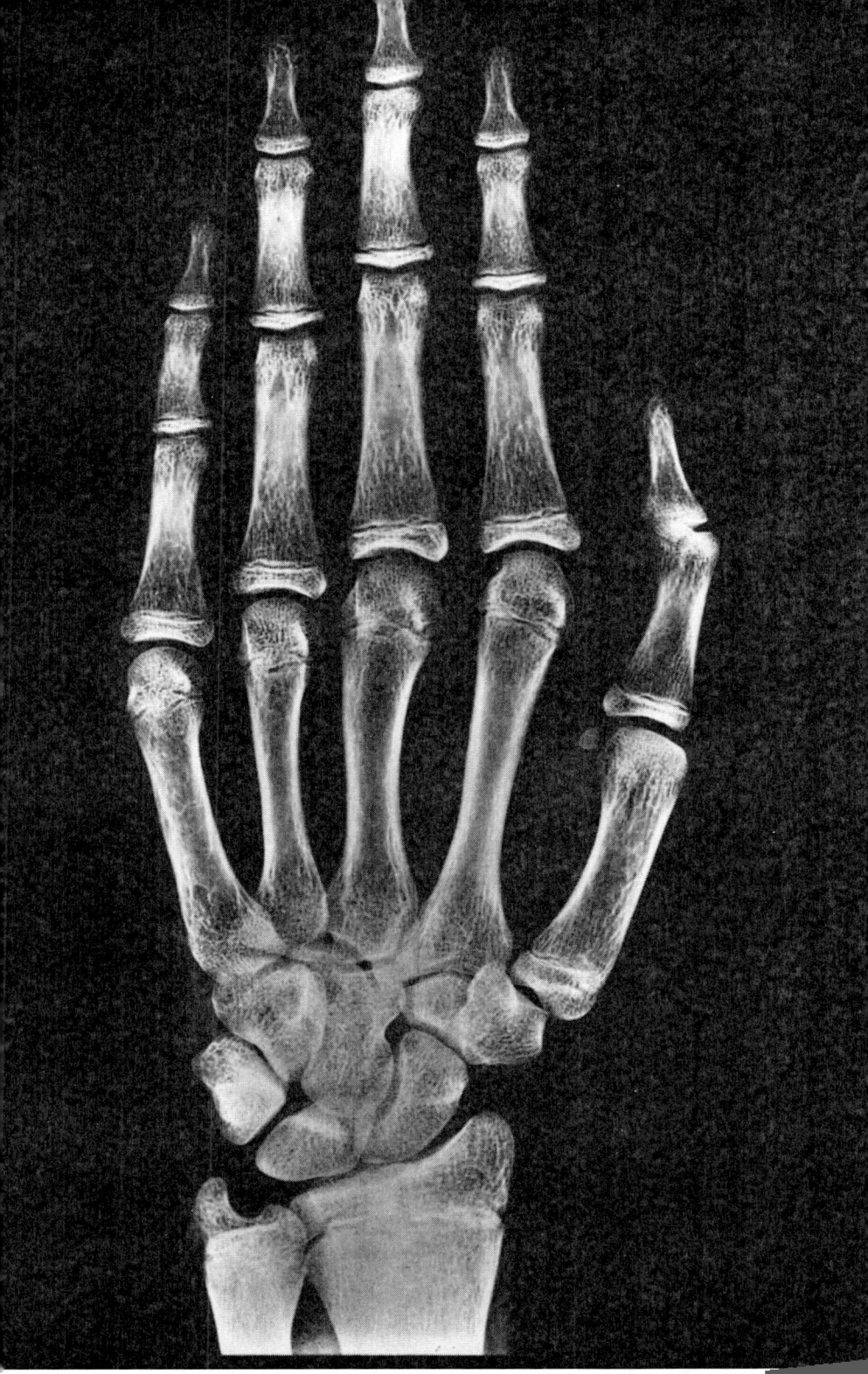

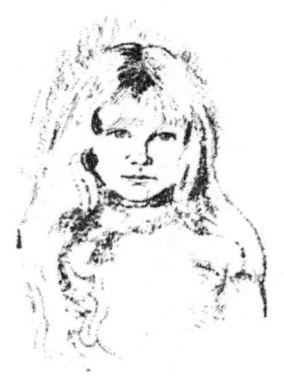

♀ 15 years

Radius and ulna: The radial and ulnar epiphyses have began to fuse with their shafts. This fusion has progressed further in the ulna than in the radius.

Carpal bones: No changes.

Metacarpal bones: Fusion of the epiphyses of all the metacarpals is completed.

Phalanges: Fusion is nearly completed in the proximal phalanges one and five and completed in the others.

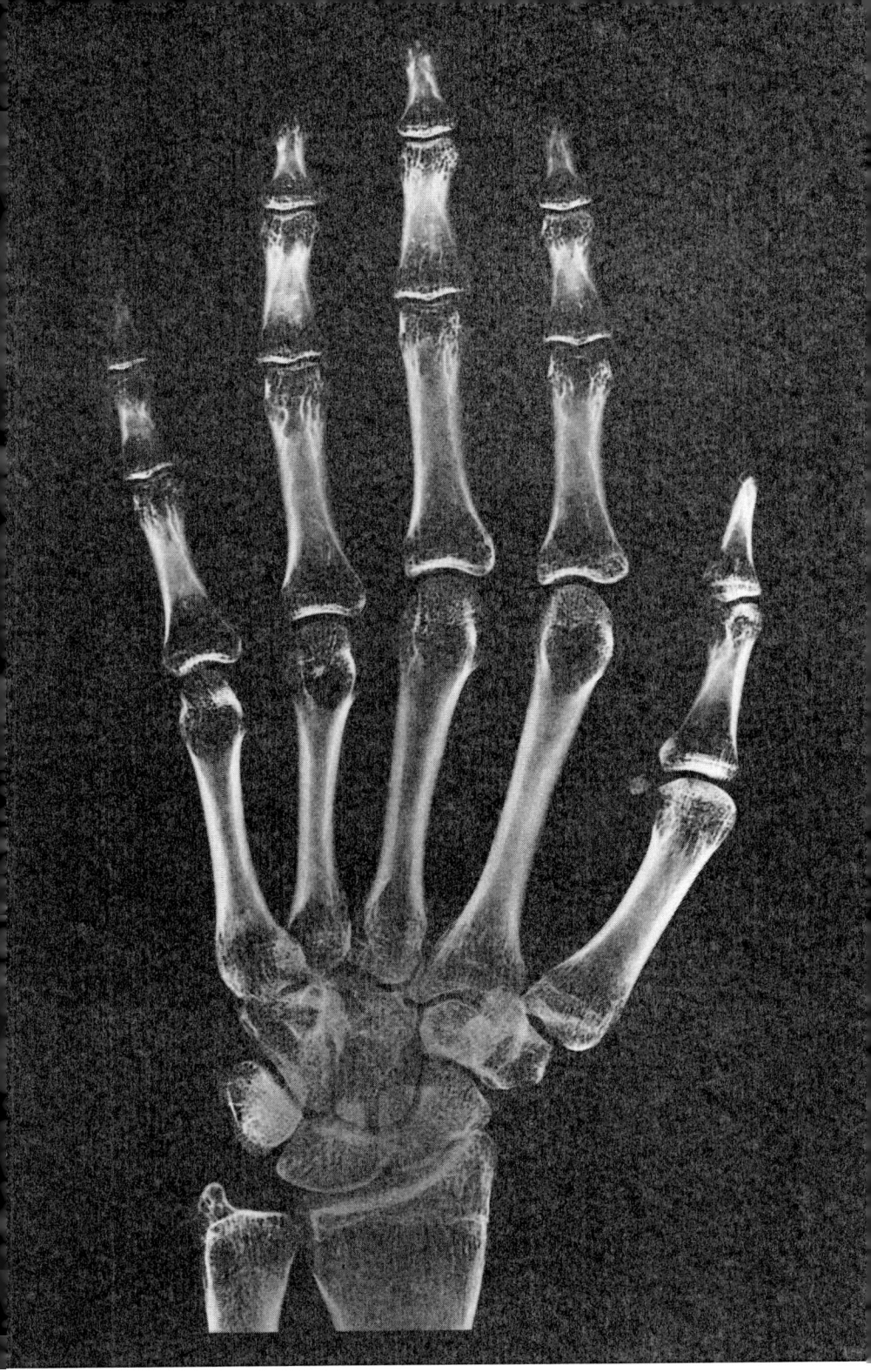

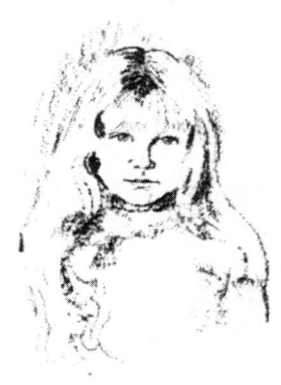

♀ 16 years

Radius and ulna: The fusion of the epiphyse of the radius has now extended to include all except the lateral margin of this junction. Fusion in the ulna is now almost complete.
Carpal bones: No changes.
Metacarpal bones: No changes.
Phalanges: No changes.

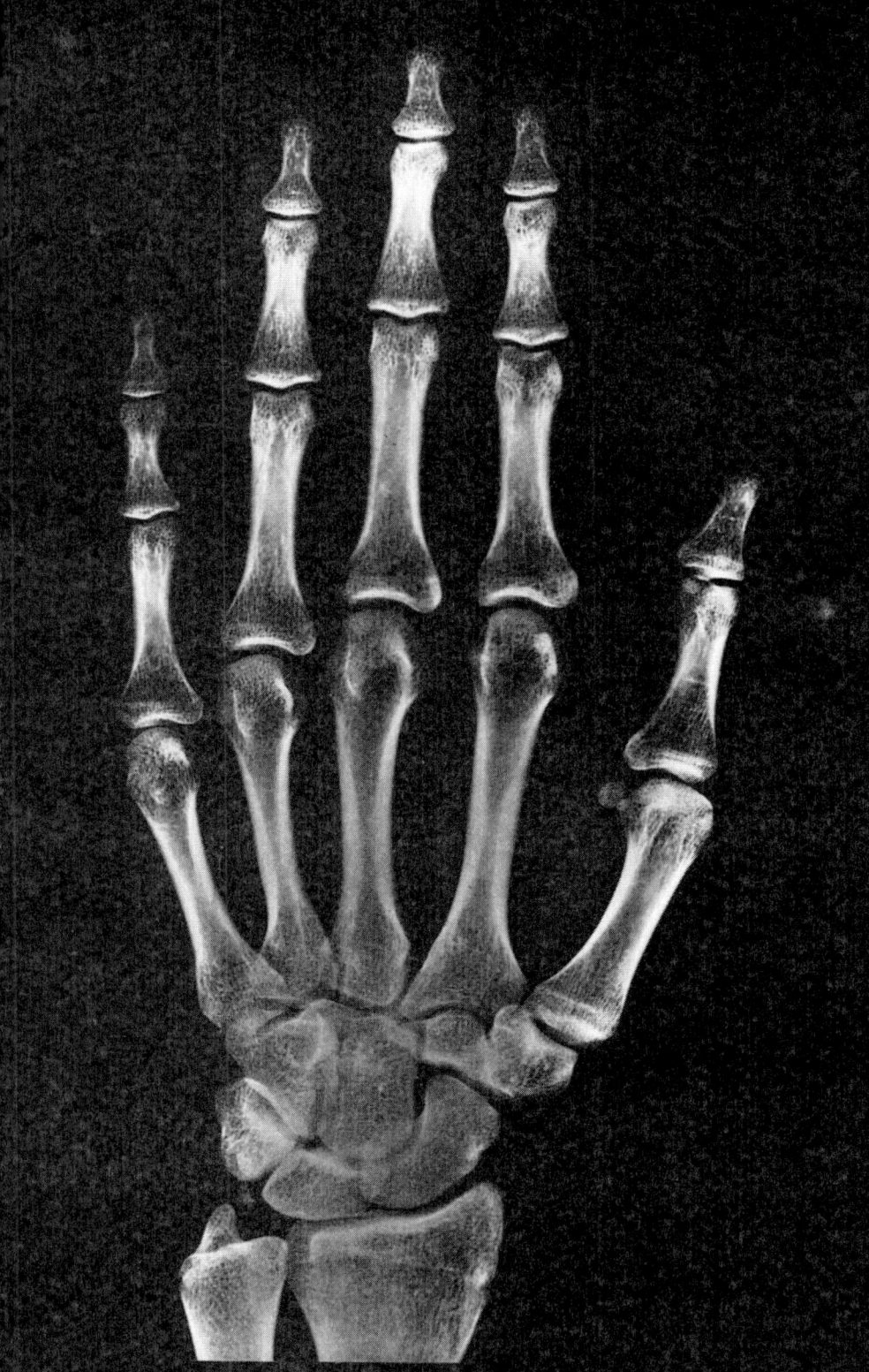

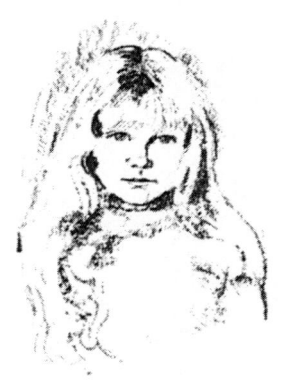

♀ 17 years

Radius and ulna: Fusion of the radius and ulna is now complete.
Carpal Bones: No changes.
Metacarpal bones: No changes.
Phalanges: The epiphyseal lines in the phalanges have almost completely obliterated.

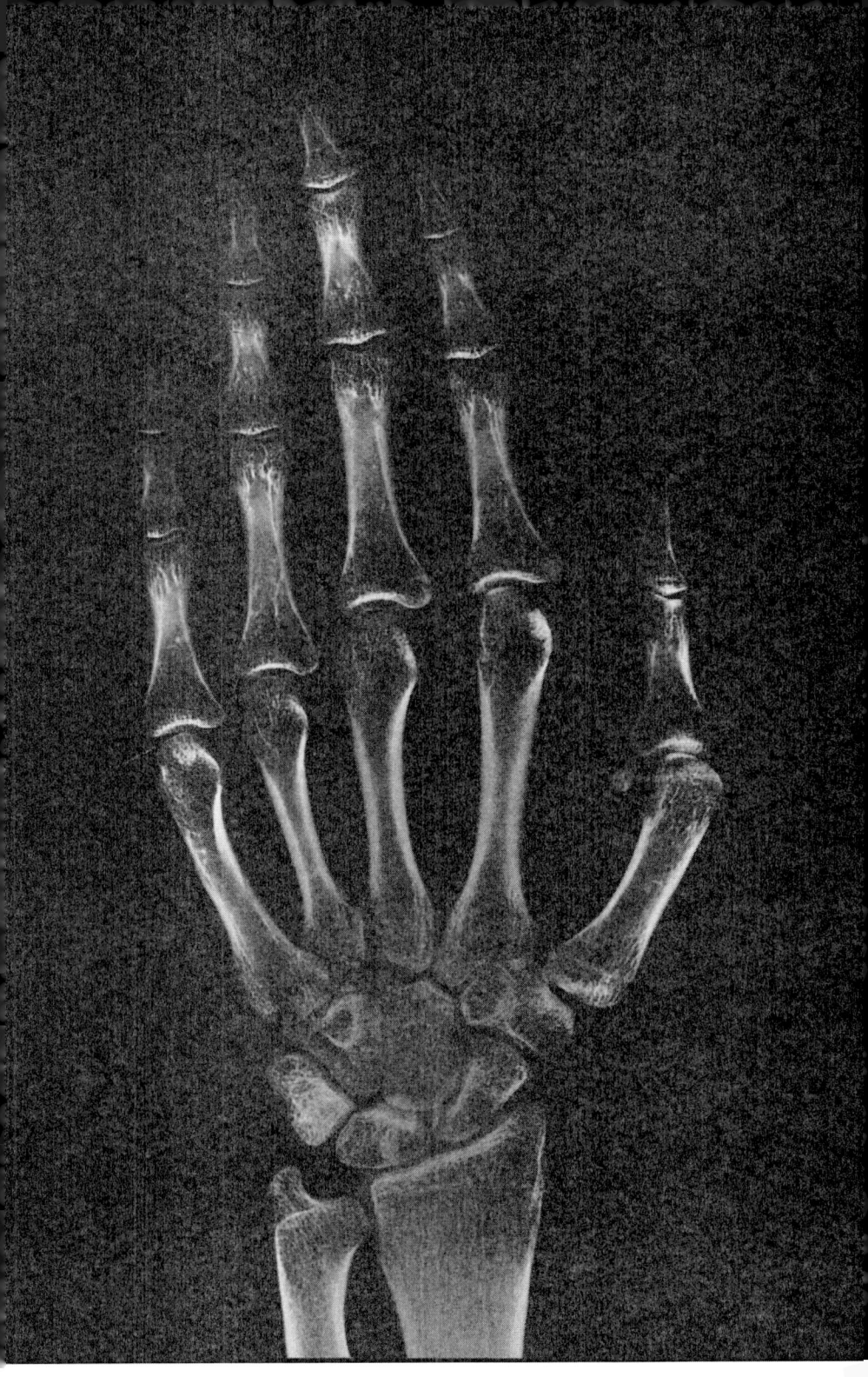

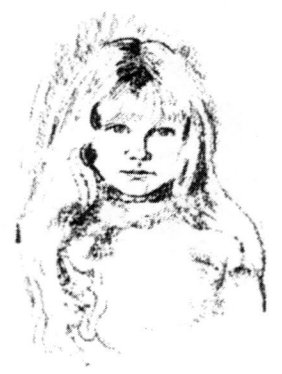

♀ 18 years

This hand is indistinguishable from that of a young adult. Traces of some epiphysial lines of fusion can still be seen.

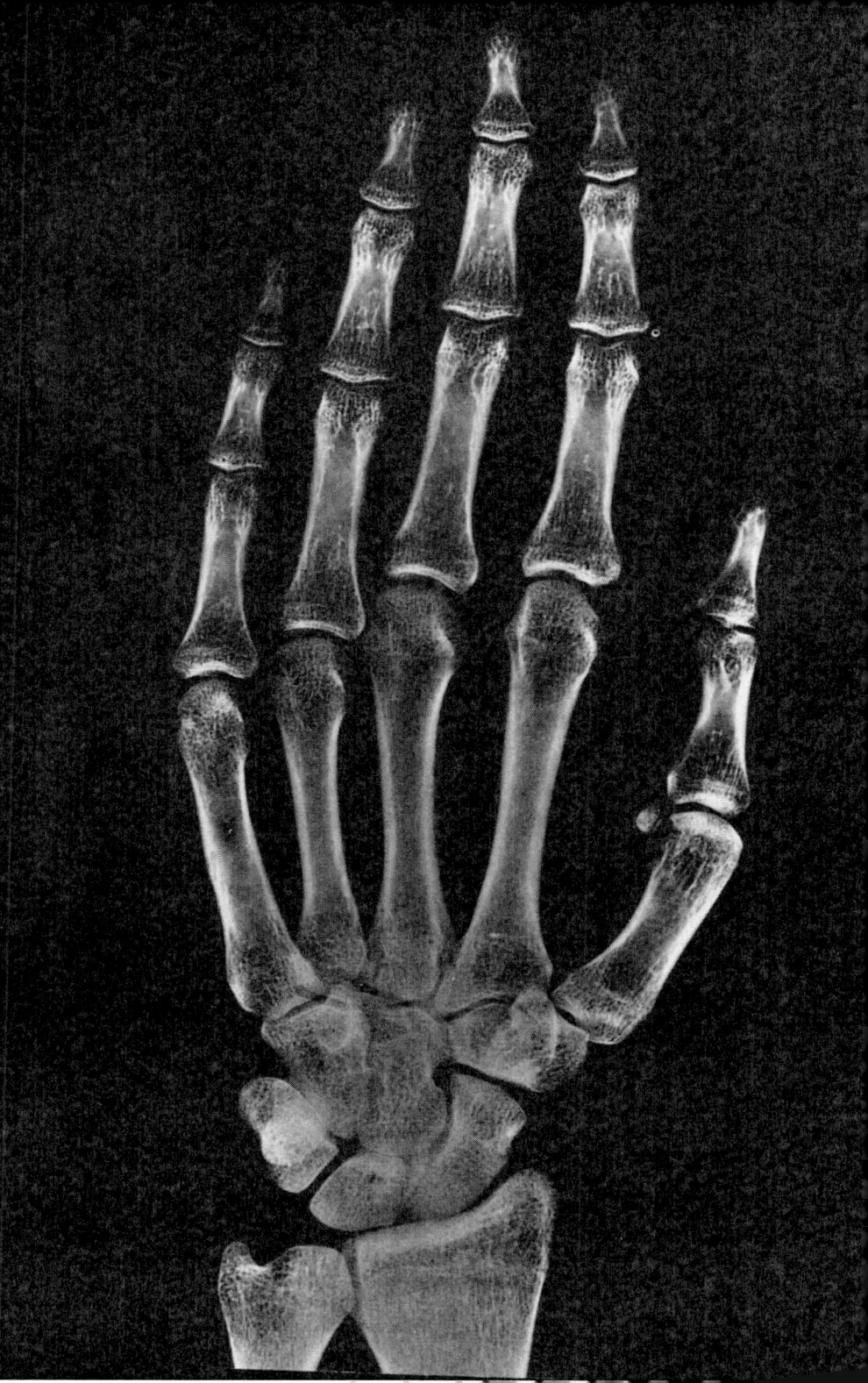